NATURE CURE
Healing Without Drugs

GW00703315

Published by
Sterling Publishers Private Limited

NATURE CURE
Healing Without Drugs

 Jindal Naturecure Institute

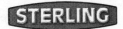

STERLING PAPERBACKS
An imprint of
Sterling Publishers (P) Ltd.
Regd. Office: A-59, Okhla Industrial Area, Phase-II,
New Delhi-110020. CIN: U22110PB1964PTC002569
Tel: 26387070, 26386209; Fax: 91-11-26383788
E-mail: mail@sterlingpublishers.com
www.sterlingpublishers.com

JINDAL NATURECURE INSTITUTE
Jindal Nagar, Tumkur Road, Bangalore 560073
Ph: 080-23717777 Fax No. 080-23717785
Email: inys@satyam.net.in
Website: http://www.naturecure-inys.org

Nature Cure: Healing Without Drugs
© 2015, Jindal Naturecure Institute, Bangalore
ISBN 978 81 207 2447 1
First Edition 2002
Reprint 2005, 2008, 2009, 2010, 2011, 2012, 2015

Printed in India

Printed and Published by Sterling Publishers Pvt. Ltd.,
New Delhi-110 020.

Contents

Foreword   xi

PART I

NATURE CURE TREATMENTS   1

I   **COMPRESSES AND FOMENTATION**   4
    COLD COMPRESS
      Abdominal Cold Compress

    HEATING COMPRESS
        Chest Pack • Abdominal Pack • Wet Girdle Pack • Throat
        Pack • Knee Pack
    HOT AND COLD COMPRESSES
        Hot and Cold Head Compress • Hot and Cold Lung
        Compress • Hot and Cold Kidney Compress • Hot and
        Cold Gastro-Hepatic Compress • Hot and Cold Pelvic
        Compress • Hot and Cold Alternate Compress on
        Abdomen
    FOMENTATION

II **BATHS**   15
    HIP BATH
        Cold Hip Bath • Neutral Hip Bath • Hot Hip Bath •
        Repulsive Hip Bath (Alternative Hip Bath) • Kuhne's
        Friction Sitz Bath
    SPINAL BATH
        Cold Spinal Bath • Neutral Spinal Bath • Hot Spinal Bath
    FOOT AND ARM BATH
        Cold Foot Bath • Hot Foot Bath • Arm Bath • Hot Foot
        and Arm Bath Combined • Contrast Arm Bath • Contrast
        Foot Bath
    STEAM INHALATION

STEAM BATH
SAUNA BATH
SPONGE BATH

III JET SPRAY MASSAGES   29
JET SPRAY MASSAGE
  Cold Jet Spray Massage • Neutral Jet Spray Massage •
  Hot Jet Spray Massage • Alternate Jet Spray Massage •
  Circular Jet Spray Massage
AFFUSION BATHS
  Cold Affusion • Neutral Affusion • Hot Affusion • Hot
  and Cold Affusion
COLD SHOWER
TROMA

IV IMMERSION BATHS   36
IMMERSION BATH
  Cold Immersion Bath • Cold Immersion Bath with
  Friction • Neutral Immersion Bath • Hot Immersion Bath
  • Neutral Half Bath • Graduated Immersion Bath with
  Epsom Salt
ASTHMA BATH
WHIRLPOOL BATH
UNDERWATER PRESSURE MASSAGE
Cold Underwater Massage • Neutral Underwater Massage

V ENEMA   46
ENEMA
  Graduated Enema
VAGINAL IRRIGATION
  Cold Irrigation • Neutral Irrigation • Hot Irrigation

VI MUD THERAPY   49
MUDPACK (LOCAL APPLICATION)
MUDPACK FOR FACE
MUDPACK FOR EYES
MUDBATH

VII MASSAGE   52
OIL MASSAGE
VIBRO-MASSAGE
COLD FRICTION
ICE MASSAGE TO HEAD AND SPINE

VIII PHYSIOTHERAPY   56
    SONOPULS
    ENDOMED
    TRANSCUTANEOUS ELECTRICAL NERVE
    STIMULATOR (TENS)
    CERVICAL AND LUMBAR INTERMITTENT
    TRACTIONS
    MILL TRAC COMPUTER
    WAX BATH
    MYO-MATIC
    VASOTRAIN
    LASER THERAPY

IX DIET   61
    DIET

PART II

DISEASES AND THEIR TREATMENTS   63

**X NUTRITION AND METABOLIC
DISORDERS**   64
    OBESITY
    DIABETES MELLITUS

**XI DISORDERS OF THE MUSCULO-SKELETAL
SYSTEM**   69
    OSTEOARTHRITIS
      Osteoarthritis of the Knee and Ankle Joints
    RHEUMATOID ARTHRITIS
    GOUTY ARTHRITIS
    ARTHRITIS OF THE SHOULDER
    SPINAL PROBLEMS
      Cervical Spondylosis • Low Backache • Ankylosing
      Spondylitis
    CALCANEAL SPUR

XII DIGESTIVE DISEASES   80
    HYPERACIDITY
    ULCERS
    FLATULENT DYSPEPSIA
    GASTRITIS
    DISORDERS OF THE SMALL INTESTINE
      Duodenitis

DISORDERS OF THE LARGE INTESTINE
   Colitis • Diverticulitis

DIARRHOEA
   Chronic Amoebiasis • Constipation

XIII   **RESPIRATORY DISEASES**   **90**
COMMON COLD
ALLERGIC RHINITIS (HAY FEVER)
RECURRENT LARYNGITIS, TONSILLITIS
SINUSITIS
BRONCHITIS
   Acute Bronchitis • Chronic Bronchitis • Asthma

XIV   **CARDIOVASCULAR SYSTEM DISEASES**   **97**
HYPERTENSION
VARICOSE VEINS

XV   **MENSTRUAL DISORDERS**   **101**
PATTERNS OF ABNORMAL UTERINE BLEEDING
PREMENSTRUAL SYNDROME (PMS)
DYSMENORRHOEA
   Primary Dysmenorrhoea • Secondary Dysmenorrhoea
LEUCORRHOEA

XVI   **URO-GENITAL DISORDERS**   **105**
THE URINARY TRACT
   Urinary Symptoms
URINARY TRACT INFECTION (UTI)
PROSTATE GLAND ENLARGEMENT

XVII   **THE NERVOUS SYSTEM DISORDERS**   **108**
INSOMNIA
HEADACHE
MIGRAINE

XVIII   **STRESS AND TENSION**   **113**

XIX   **COLON HYDROTHERAPY**   **115**

XX   **ACUPUNCTURE**   **117**

XXI   **MISCELLANEOUS CONDITIONS**   **119**
FEVER
ABSCESSES

BUNIONS
BRUISES, STRAINS, SPRAINS AND MUSCLE
INJURIES
HEAT EXHAUSTION
HICCOUGH
EPISTAXIS (NOSEBLEEDING)
TOOTHACHE

XXII **TIPS FOR HEALTHY LIVING**   **124**
MAINTAIN
   Water • Vital Factors • Rest • Exercise • Food
REDUCE/MODERATE
AVOID
PRACTISE
PRECAUTIONS
ADOPT
POINTS TO REMEMBER
POINTS AT A GLANCE

Glossary   **129**

Foreword

This book is designed to help the reader understand the principles of the healing science of nature cure and its treatment modalities. Nature is the best healer and naturopathy or nature cure is the adoption of nature's own tools, the five great elements—Earth, Water, Air, Fire and Space—to cure the diseases that afflict mankind.

Many diseases can be avoided by following healthy habits, taking good, nutritious food and doing proper exercises. But if diseases strike despite all these precautions, it is better to cure them by following the edicts of nature cure and yoga. Another advantage of nature cure is that it is a drugless therapy and, hence, free from any ill-effects of chemicals.

This book is a humble attempt of the *Jindal Naturecure Institute (JNI)* to consolidate and systematise some of the natural methods known for curing diseases, including yoga, which, too, is a drugless therapy.

Efforts have keen made to make the book more objective and useful by giving the details of the treatments and application vis-à-vis the diseases.

This book is meant for all those who seek to cure their ailments through nature cure methods. However, scrupulous care must be taken in the use of these methods and patients must guard against their misapplication.

Patients are advised to read the treatment methods carefully before adopting them. If these are not immediately clear, they are advised to consult a naturopath for guidance.

Yoga, the ancient method of exercise and relaxation, forms another successful method of preventing and curing diseases. The study and research at the JNI vouchsafe this unassailable fact. It is aptly said, "Nature cure and yoga are the two wheels of a cart on the road to a healthier life."

JNI has published many books earlier, on various subjects of naturopathy, yoga and diet. This book is yet another attempt to enlighten and ensure for the ailing mankind, a healthier life.

B.V. Garg
Chairman, INYS

Nature Cure Treatments

PREAMBLE

The Institute of Naturopathy and Yogic Sciences (a charitable hospital) believes that the first step in curing a patient is in educating him about the system of nature cure and yoga, as when the patient is fully aware of the treatments prescribed, he extends his cooperation and reaps rich benefits.

This book is intended to explain and guide the patient about the various methods of treatments adopted in the Institute. It also briefs them about their benefits. Patients are, therefore, requested to go through this book carefully. Better results could be achieved by following the treatments as prescribed.

The following points should be kept in mind while undergoing treatment.

GENERAL RULES

1. At least two litres of water should be taken every day.

2. The interval between meals and the treatments should be at least three hours after eating and at least one hour before it. Only in exceptional circumstances and on doctor's advice, the rule can be relaxed.

3. Clean and pure water must be used for treatments.

4. Water once used for any treatment should not be reused.

5. Linen and packs should be thoroughly washed in hot water and dried before they are used for treatment.

6. The treatment rooms should be well-ventilated, clean and comfortably warm. Direct exposure to breeze should be prevented while the patient is undergoing treatment.

1

7. Very weak patients and patients suffering from heart disease, high blood pressure, fever or extreme exhaustion should not take prolonged hot or cold water treatments, steam and sauna baths. If prescribed by the doctor, they should take these under the supervision of a trained nurse.

8. While undergoing hydropathic treatments, the temperature and duration of the application should be strictly observed to obtain the desired effects. Unnecessary prolonging the treatment in the belief of securing better result is, in fact, harmful.

9. Before and after taking cold water treatments, patients should not walk barefoot on wet ground or wet grass and should not be exposed to cold air. They should wear slippers to protect their feet.

10. After cold water treatments, patients should quickly dry themselves and undertake moderate exercises such as yogasanas, suryanamaskaras, pranayama, etc. If the patients are not in a position to do asanas or exercise, they are advised to take a brisk walk for twenty minutes. If they are too weak to do even that, they should cover themselves with a blanket until the reaction of the treatment wears off (about thirty minutes).

11. Cold water treatments should be discontinued immediately if the patient feels chill. Even a second more may cause him nausea, giddiness, etc. Sometimes, this may also cause a condition known as Hydrotherapic Fever.

12. After cold water treatments, bath should be taken only after an interval of thirty to forty-five minutes.

13. While taking hot water treatments, necessary precautions mentioned in the concerned treatment procedure should be taken for better results. If they are ignored, they might prove dangerous. After taking hot water treatments, a quick cold shower is a must.

14. Before taking any hot water treatment, the patient should drink one or two glasses of cold water. The head should always be protected with a wet towel to keep the brain cool; otherwise, the patient may feel giddy, nauseous and may even faint.

Terminate the treatment as soon as the patient shows the slightest indication of giddiness or weakness/exhaustion.

15. During the menstrual period, women should not take any treatment. If necessary, they may take enema, cold water bath and other minor treatments, only on doctor's advice.

16. During pregnancy, till the completion of third month, women can take cold hip bath, and thereafter, only cold towel packs are advised. Other treatments should be taken only under a doctor's guidance.

17. Sometimes, during the treatment, a healing crisis may occur. It generally consists of aggravation of the disease, fever, skin trouble, Diarrhoea, Dysentery, etc. In such cases, one need not be alarmed, since it is nothing but a vigorous action of the body to eliminate the disease-producing morbid matter. During the period of crisis, treatment and diet should be strictly adhered to and complete bed-rest taken. The body will be relieved of all unwanted morbid matter and get revitalised and rejuvenated soon.

Chapter I

Compresses and Fomentation

COLD COMPRESS

Cold compress is a local, cold application by means of a cloth dipped in cold water.

Requisites: Two thick cotton or linen cloths or large towels.

Water Temperature: Cold water, 18 to 24°C, or ice water, 0°C, wherever indicated.

Duration: Twenty minutes. May be prolonged in some conditions.

Procedure: The cloth should be folded into four folds and dipped in cold water. Before application, it should be wrung well and applied on the concerned part of the body. When the compress is applied continuously, it should be renewed frequently by using two compresses alternately. The compress can be applied to the head, neck, chest, abdomen, spine or on any inflamed portion of the body. When applied on the head, it should be pressed firmly so that it is in contact with the scalp. The pillow should be covered with a rubber sheet and towel. Similarly, when applied to the abdomen, the patient's bedding should be covered suitably.

Uses: Cold compress is used to regulate the blood circulation and functions of the liver, spleen, stomach, kidneys, intestines, lungs, brain, uterus, bladder and other internal organs. It is used to control inflammatory conditions of these organs.

The cold compress is valuable in treating localised inflammatory conditions, whether superficial or deep.

It can be advantageously employed in cases of fever. Repeated application of the cold compress on the head lowers the temperature. The cold compress applied over the area of the heart reduces palpitation and also helps in lowering the temperature of the blood as it passes through the heart and lungs. Cold compress over the face and the upper spine stops nose bleeding. This also helps stop bleeding in case of Piles and Haemorrhage in the above mentioned organs.

It can also be applied by using an ice bag to stop bleeding in any internal organ and from external wounds. In case of severe vomiting, the ice bag may be applied over the stomach.

The cold compress cools the skin in Dermatitis and relieves inflammation of external portions of the eye. When the eye ball is affected, the cold compress should be applied after a short fomentation.

Abdominal Cold Compress (Cold Towel Pack)
Procedure: Dip a towel in cold water and wring it to remove excess water. Fold the towel into three or four folds to make it twelve to fourteen inches long and ten inches wide. Place it on the abdomen,

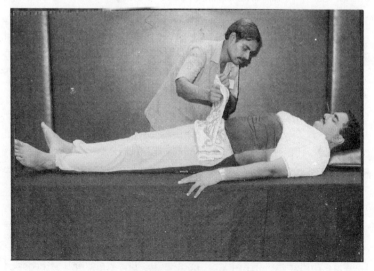

Cold Towel Pack

covering it with another dry towel or woollen cloth. After ten minutes, reverse the towel so that the top portion touches the abdomen and leave it there for another ten minutes. If necessary, repeat the process for a longer time by dipping the towel again in cold water.

Uses: It increases the blood circulation to the abdominal organs, activates metabolic functions, reduces inflammation and calms the nervous system. It produces a feeling of comfort and relieves pain and congestion in digestive, reproductive and urinary organs.

HEATING COMPRESS

The heating compress is a cold compress covered up in such a manner that warming occurs soon. The effect is that of a mild application of moist heat. A heating compress consists of three or four folds of linen cloth dipped in cold water, wrung out and covered completely with a dry cloth and a flannel or a blanket to prevent circulation of air and help accumulation of body heat. The duration of the application is minimum one hour, but sometimes can be extended to several hours. If applied at night and the patient falls asleep, he/she should not be disturbed. After removing the compress, the area should be rubbed with a wet cloth and dried with a towel.

The heating compress can be applied to the throat (throat compress), chest (chest compress/chest pack), abdomen (abdomen compress), joints (joints compress) and so on. In all the compresses mentioned below, the water used is cold.

Chest Compress or Chest Pack

Requisites: Two cotton chest compresses and a blanket or a flannel compress. The size of the compress should be two to two-and-a-half metres long and about half a metre wide, depending upon the size of the chest of the patient.

Duration: One hour.

Procedure: A cotton compress is dipped in cold water and wrung out. The cloth is placed on the back and the two ends are brought forward under the armpits on each side. The right half is crossed over the left shoulder and the left part over the end, across the right shoulder. Both are again crossed at the back and the ends are brought forward under the armpits and tucked in at the front. Cover this with a dry cloth and then with a flannel. The pack should be as comfortably tight as possible.

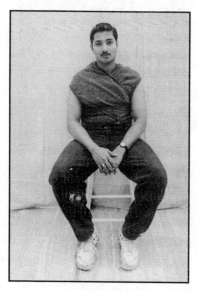

Chest Pack

Uses: Since this application will have very soothing effect, most of the patients fall asleep within minutes. They should not be disturbed.

It is helpful in relieving Cold, Bronchitis, Asthma, Pleurisy, Pneumonia, Fever, Cough, Whooping Cough, etc.

Abdominal Pack
Requisites: Two cotton cloths of two to two-and-a-half metres length and half a metre width. Blanket or flannel, one by half metre.

Duration: One hour.

Procedure: Dip the cotton cloth in cold water and wring out to remove the excess water. Wrap the cloth around the abdomen from lower part of the ribs to the groin. Over this, wrap the dry cloth, and finally, the flannel so that the pack fits snugly.

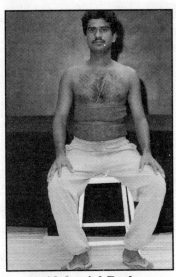

Abdomial Pack

Uses: Abdominal compress is useful in cases of Gastritis, Hyperacidity, Indigestion, poor blood circulation to the liver, Jaundice, Constipation and other complaints relating to the abdominal organs.

Wet Girdle Pack

Requisites: Two pairs of underwear, one made of cotton and the other of thick cotton or, preferably, woollen.

Duration: One hour.

Procedure: The underwear should cover the whole pelvic girdle. The patient should wear the thin, cotton underwear wrung in cold water and the thicker one over it.

Uses: It is useful in treating all pelvic and genito-urinary problems, specifically the following diseases: Dysmenorrhoea (painful menstruation), Menorrhagia (excessive menstruation), Leucorrhoea (white discharge), Recurring Appendicitis, Urinary Incontinence, Burning Micturation, Urinary Tract Infection, Bleeding Piles, Bleeding Fibroid of the uterus, and in all acute pelvic inflammations and congestion.

Throat Pack
Requisites: Two cotton cloths (one dipped in cold water, the other dry) and a flannel, each six feet long, five inches wide.

Procedure: Wrap the cold cloth around the neck in several layers and, on that, the dry cloth, like in any other pack. Finally, the dry flannel.

Duration: One hour.

Uses: Throat compress is useful in treating sore throat, hoarseness, Tonsillitis, Pharyngitis, Laryngitis, inflammation of the Eustachian tubes, etc.

Knee Pack
Requisites: Materials as used in throat pack.

Duration: One hour.

Uses: The knee joint compress is helpful in treating inflammed knees and is useful in Arthritis, to relieve pain and stiffness.

HOT AND COLD COMPRESSES
In this treatment, hot and cold applications are made to stimulate the skin surface colaterally related to an internal part. This unique treatment is applicable under appropriate conditions, only to head, chest, spine, abdomen and pelvis. It helps in treating all types of muscular pains and spasms.

The duration of treatment by hot and cold compress may extend from fifteen minutes to forty five minutes or until the desired effect is obtained. The application relieves congestion in internal organs. This is one of the most powerful hydriatic measures.

Hot and Cold Head Compress
Requisites: Ice bag, two compresses—one ice-cold, one hot.

Water Temperature: Ice-cold water, 0°C, hot water, 42 to 45°C.

Duration: Fifteen to forty-five minutes.

Procedure: Place the ice bag filled with ice-cold water at the back of the neck and ice compress at the back of the head. Apply very hot compress to the face and ears. The hot compress should not extend below the jaw line, in order to avoid heating of the blood vessels of the neck. The cold compress at the back of the head causes reflex contraction of the vessels of the brain and cools it. The fomentation draws blood from the brain to the facial muscles. The same method may be applied inversely, as follows:

A rubber bag filled with hot water and covered with a moist cloth is applied over the upper back part of the neck, while the cold compress is applied to the face and the top of the head. The effect of this compress is to relieve the congestion of the brain.

Uses: In most of the headaches, especially those due to irritability of the cranial nerves (especially eye and ear nerves), this application forms a valuable treatment. It induces sleep and thus helps in curing Insomnia.

Contraindication: In headaches caused by Anaemia.

Hot and Cold Lung Compress

Requisites: Hot water bag, cold compress.

Water Temperature: Cold, 18 to 25°C, hot, 42 to 45°C.

Duration: Fifteen to forty-five minutes.

Procedure: The hot water bag is applied to the back and cold application is made over the lungs, extending from the lower half of the neck in the front, upto the lowest rib. The fomentation diverts the blood from the arteries of the lungs, dilating the blood vessels of the intercostals, while the cold compress contracts the arteries of the lungs. This effect can be improved by hot bath or hot pack given to the legs at the same time.

Uses: This application is useful in treating the earlier stages of Pneumonia and acute congestion in the lungs.

In cases of Asthma, the procedure has to be reversed. Ice compress is to be applied on the back of the neck and head while the fomentation is to be applied over the whole front part of the chest, extending from the collar bone to the umbilicus. Later, the fomentation may be extended to the back.

Hot and Cold Kidney Compress

Requisites: Hot water bag, ice bag, and other material as for abdomen pack.

Water Temperature: Hot water, 42 to 45°C, ice-cold water.

Duration: Forty-five minutes.

Procedure: The flannel and dry cloth of the abdomen pack are spread out on the table or bed. The hot water bag is placed on this and the patient is made to lie down in such a way that the hot water bag extends from the mid spine to the lower spine. The ice bag is placed on the abdomen, extending upto the lower portion of the chest bone (sternum). The abdomen pack is wrapped over this.

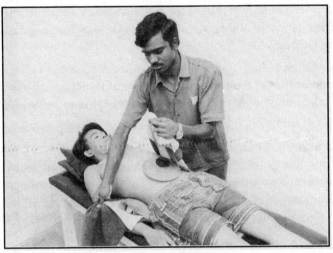

Kidney Compress

Uses: Fomentation diverts the blood from the branches of the renal artery, which is connected to the kidney, and leads off a portion of it from the renal vein into the muscular branches. The cold application causes contraction of the blood vessels of the kidney and thereby increases its activity. This pack is useful in cases of acute congestion of the kidney and inflammation of the urinary tract. It strengthens the kidney and, hence, is useful in Albuminuria

11

(albumin outflow with urine), burning urination and stones in the kidney. This pack increases the output of urine.

Hot and Cold Gastro-Hepatic Compress

Requisites, water temperature and *duration* as of kidney pack.

Procedure: This application is exactly the reverse of the kidney compress. Fomentation bag should be applied to the abdominal region, covering the area from the fourth rib to the umbilicus, while the cold application is made to the middle and lower spine.

Uses: During this application, the blood is drained from the stomach, liver, spleen and pancreas and congestion is relieved. Thus, this pack influences not only the stomach and liver, but also the spleen and the pancreas. It is helpful in cases of Gastritis, liver and spleen enlargement, ulcers in the stomach, Hyperacidity and inflammation of the pancreas. This pack is extensively used to treat Diabetes Mellitus.

Precautions: It is found that blood pressure tends to increase temporarily after this pack, hence, in case of Hypertension, it should be taken only under a doctor's guidance. It is to be avoided in cases of mid and lower back pain.

Hot and Cold Pelvic Compress

In this, the cold compress is applied over the lower back and fomentation over the pelvic region. This is useful in treating acute inflammation of the uterus, fallopian tubes, ovaries, bladder, prostate, testicles and appendix.

Hot and Cold Alternate Compress on Abdomen

Requisites: Two pieces of khaddar or towel-type cloth, folded into six or eight layers.

Water Temperature: Tolerable warm water, cold tap water.

Procedure: Soak a piece of cloth in warm water and after wringing out the excess water, keep the cloth on the abdomen for three minutes. To maintain the cloth's warmth, place a hot water bag or another cloth soaked in warm water on it. After three minutes, remove it and keep a cloth soaked in cold water over the abdomen for only one minute. Repeat this alternate process three times, but the last cold compress should be for three minutes.

On the advice of the naturopath, the treatment can be varied by keeping warm compress for five minutes and cold for two minutes, alternately.

Uses: This treatment is given for relieving gastro-intestinal gases, Hyperacidity, Constipation and to increase secretion of gastric juices, to relieve congestion in liver and gall bladder.

Contraindication: This treatment can be given on any painful part of the body, except the heart.

Note: During summer, when ordinary water is not cold, ice water or water stored in earthen pots overnight, preferably on the terrace of the house, can be used for cold compress.

FOMENTATION

Requisites: Hot water bag or cotton cloth wrung in hot water, a cold compress and a dry cloth.

Water Temperature: 42 to 45°C.

Duration: Five to seven minutes.

Procedure: When the hot water bag is used, it is advisable to cover the area of application with a cotton cloth wrung in cold water. Fomentation is then applied over it. After the application is over, a cloth dipped in cold water should be placed on the same area for one to two minutes. After removing the wet cloth, it should be covered with a dry cloth for at least thirty to forty minutes. If the symptoms recur, the application should be renewed.

Uses: For relieving acute pain in any part of the body, especially in the abdomen, it is an invaluable treatment. In arthritic pains, this may be repeated twice or thrice a day for better results. In cases like Bronchitis, Asthma, Pneumonia, Pleurisy, fomentation to the upper back gives immediate relief. In congestive headaches, fomentation should be applied over the back of the neck and shoulders, and the face washed with very cold water. Fomentation is used to relieve both the pain and the congestion in cases of inflammation of liver, acute and chronic Gastritis, splenic congestion and enlargement, inflammation of the ovaries and uterus and other muscular pains. It also helps to relieve pain caused due to Gallstones, Kidney-stones, infection, Jaundice, etc. When the patient feels extremely cold, he may be given fomentation over the whole back and to the feet and hands. Within ten to fifteen minutes, he will get relief. In inflammatory conditions like Diphtheria, Tonsillitis and throat pain caused due to cold, fomentation given on the throat gives immense relief. It is also helpful in menstrual pains associated with scanty flow. It may be given on the perineum in case of prostatic inflammation. In urine retention, fomentation may be given over the lower abdomen for ten minutes, followed by cold friction for one minute. In Bell's Palsy, fomentation to the facial muscles will improve the condition.

Precautions and contraindications:

1. The temperature of water should be only as high as bearable.

2. Fomentation should not be overdone as it causes damage to the skin tissues. While giving fomentation in neuralgia, care should be taken to not to burn the skin.

3. Fomentation should be avoided on the heart, head and on the seat of active inflammation (open wound).

4. It should not be given over the abdomen in advanced pregnancy and during menstruation period, unless advised otherwise by the doctor.

Chapter II

Baths

HIP BATH
Hip bath is given at cold, neutral, hot and alternate temperatures in a special hip bathtub.

Cold Hip Bath
Requisites: Hip bathtub, a moderately coarse cloth (the size of a handkerchief).

Water Temperature: Cold, 18 to 24°C.

Duration: Fifteen minutes, unless otherwise indicated.

Procedure: The tub should be filled with cold water, enough to cover the hips and reaching upto the navel of the patient, when he sits in it. Generally, four to six gallons of water are necessary. If

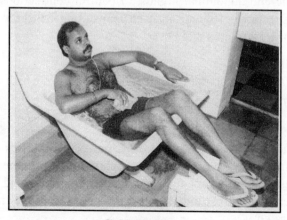

Cold Hip Bath

15

the patient feels chill or when the climate is very cold or if the patient is very weak, a hot foot bath should be given along with the cold hip bath.

The patient should gently rub the abdomen, around the navel, in clockwise direction, with the coarse, wet cloth. This should be continued during the entire period of the bath. It is important that the legs, feet and the upper part of the body are thoroughly dry and do not get wet during and after the bath. Wear shoes before entering the bath. After the cold hip bath, the patient should undertake moderate exercises like brisk walking, yogasanas, suryanamaskaras, etc. If he is very weak, he should lie down in bed and be covered with a blanket.

Uses: A cold hip bath is a routine treatment for almost all diseases. The treatment is meant to relieve Constipation, Indigestion, Obesity and to help the eliminative organs to function properly. This bath is also helpful in subinvolution of the uterus, inflammation of the pelvic organs, Piles, hepatic and splenic congestion, Urinary Incontinence in young children, chronic uterine infections, chronic congestion of the prostate, seminal weakness, atony of bladder in both sexes, impotency, sterility, and dilation of the stomach and colon.

Contraindication: Avoid in cases of inflammation and neuralgias of pelvic and abdominal organs, in painful contractions of the bladder, rectum or vagina, low back pain, during menstrual period, Diarrhoea, Dysentery and Fever.

Neutral Hip Bath
Requisities: Cold compress for the head, besides the bath tub.

Water Temperature: 32 to 36°C.

Duration: Fifteen minutes.

Procedure: The patient should drink one or two glasses of cold water and sit in the tub, avoiding friction to the abdomen. Cold compress should be kept on the head. After bath, both cold shower and exercise are to be avoided. Relaxation/rest for thirty minutes is advocated.

Uses: The neutral hip bath is helpful in relieving all acute and sub-acute inflammatory conditions of the bladder and urethra, uterus, ovaries and fallopian tubes. It helps in relieving neuralgia of the fallopian tubes, testicles, painful spasm of the vagina, pruritus (itching) of the anus and vulva, and hyperaesthesia (excessive sensitivity) of the abdominal organs. It is a sedative treatment for Erotomania in both sexes and an ideal one for Spermatorrhoea.

Hot Hip Bath

Requisites: Hip bathtub, one cold compress.

Water Temperature: 40 to 45°C.

Duration: Ten minutes.

Procedure: The patient should drink one or two glasses of cold water before the treatment. The bath should start with water at 40°C and the temperature be increased gradually, to the required level. Its temperature should be maintained by adding either hot or cold water. While undergoing the hot hip bath, the patient should not apply friction to the abdomen. During the treatment, a cold compress should be placed over his head. Thereafter, the patient should take a cold water shower for one or two minutes.

Uses: Hot hip bath is used in cases of delayed menstruation, pain in the pelvic organs, painful urination, inflammed rectum or bladder or pain due to Piles. It is also useful in cases of enlarged prostate gland, painful contractions or spasm of the bladder, Sciatica, neuralgia of the ovaries and bladder, Lumbar Spondylosis, etc. It also helps in relieving painful menstruation (but should be avoided during periods).

Contraindication: It should be avoided in case of recurrent high blood pressure, weakness and fever.

Precautions: Care should be taken to prevent the patient from catching cold after the bath as it causes unpleasant symptoms and spoils the reaction. Terminate the bath if the patient feels giddy or weak or complains of excessive pain.

Repulsive Hip Bath (Alternative Hip Bath)

Requisites: Two hip bathtubs, cold compress.

Water Temperature: Hot, 40 to 45°C, cold 18 to 24°C.

Procedure: There are two methods of giving this bath. In both the methods, one or two glasses of water should be taken before treatment. The head should be kept cool by applying a cold compress over the head. The treatment should end with cold hip bath.

1. The patient first sits in the hot tub for five minutes and then in the cold tub for five minutes. This increases the peristalitic movement of the digestive system and relieves constipation and gases. This also activates the kidney and other genito-urinary organs. It reduces irritability caused due to infections.

2. The second method of giving alternative hip bath is three minutes hot and one minute cold, repeated four to five times.

Uses: This also relieves deep-seated pain of gastric origin or pain caused due to severe Constipation. It eases the pain in the lumbar vertebrae. This bath is helpful in treating other disorders like incontinence of urine and stones in the kidney. It also helps in relieving chronic, inflammatory conditions of the pelvic organs, such as Salpingitis, Oophoritis, Cellulitis and neuralgias and hyperaesthesia of the genito-urinary organs, Sciatica, Lumbago, etc.

Kuhne's Friction Sitz Bath

This is also known as genital bath or *linga snan.*

Requisites: Hip bathtub, a stool specially made for this, a soft, linen cloth.

Water Temperature: Cold, 18 to 24°C.

Duration: Two to ten minutes.

Procedure: The stool specially made for this bath is placed in the hip bathtub. The tub is filled with cold water, leaving the top of the stool dry. The patient sits on the stool, keeping the legs outside the tub. In case of a female patient, she dips a soft, linen cloth in the water and gently washes the genitals from top, downwards. It is important that the external lips only be washed and inner parts of the sexual organs left unwashed and untouched.

In case of males, the extreme edge of the foreskin of the genitals is washed in cold water. The patient should hold the foreskin between his middle and forefinger of the left hand and draw as far as possible over tip of the glans penis, till the skin touches the water level in the tub. He should, then, gently wash the extreme end of the foreskin with a soft cloth. Under no circumstances should the cloth in the right hand touch the glans penis.

Soon after the bath, care should be taken to restore the warmth of the body by undertaking moderate exercise.

Uses: This treatment stimulates the nervous system, since the genitals are known to be an important centre of the central nervous system. In subnormal temperatures, it produces necessary heat in the body. Morbid internal heat in the body is diminished and, at the same time, a marked invigoration of the nervous system with increased vitality can be achieved by this application.

SPINAL BATH

Spinal baths are given in tubs specially made for the purpose. Like the hip bath, it is also given at cold, neutral and hot temperatures. A perforated tube is provided at the centre of the tub in order that the constantly emanating, ascending jet will give a gentle massage to the whole spinal column. This tub is not only very comfortable, but also helps to maintain constant water temperature. The gentle massage of the fine water columns is capable of giving quick results. The patient has to lie down in the tub so that the whole spinal cord receives the water columns.

Cold Spinal Bath

Water Temperature: Cold, 18 to 24°C.

Duration: Fifteen minutes.

Procedure: The patient lies in the spinal bathtub after getting undressed and adjusts himself to the water columns of the tub such that they touch the entire length of the spine—from the nape of the neck to the lowest portion of the spine. Some footwear should be worn all along so that the circulation is not interfered with. After the bath, the patient should walk briskly or perform suryanamaskaras so that heat is generated in the body. If the patient is weak, he can lie down on the bed and cover himself with a blanket.

Uses: Cold spinal bath relieves irritation of nerves, fatigue, high blood pressure and excitement. It is recommended in almost all nervous disorders, such as hysteria, fits, mental derangement, sleeplessness, loss of memory, tension, etc.

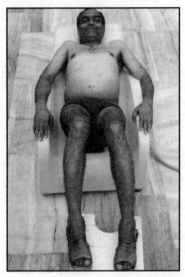

Cold Spinal Bath

Contraindication: Cervical and Lumbar Spondylosis, and Arthritis.

Neutral Spinal Bath
Water Temperature: 34 to 36°C.

Duration: Fifteen minutes.

Procedure: The patient should drink one or two glasses of cold water before the bath and keep the head cool. The procedure is same as in the cold spinal bath, except that after the bath exercise should *not* be done. Instead, the patient should relax for half an hour.

20

The neutral spinal bath is a soothing and sedative treatment, especially when the nerves are in an irritable condition. It is the ideal treatment recommended for Insomnia. It also relieves muscular tension of the vertebral column when it is exhausted with prolonged sitting, exercise and labour. It eases congestion of the lungs and relaxes the cardiac muscles.

This bath also soothes the nervous system, the back muscles, low back sprains and helps one in treating Sciatica.

Hot Spinal Bath
Water Temperature: 40 to 45°C.

Duration: Ten minutes.

Procedure: As in neutral spinal bath. All precautions recommended for the hot hip bath should be taken during this treatment.

Uses: Hot spinal bath is helpful in stimulating the nerves, especially when they are in a depressed stage. It also relieves back pain, Sciatica and gastro-intestinal disturbances.

FOOT AND ARM BATH
Foot and arm baths are intended to increase blood circulation or, if needed, lessen it. Thus, the monitored blood circulation can produce warmth, sweating or reduce the temperature of a particular body part. In these baths, either the arms or feet or both are immersed in water upto above elbows and calf muscles, respectively, while sitting on a stool.

Cold Foot Bath
Requisites: A small tub or bucket.

Water Temperature: 8 to 12°C.

Duration: One to five minutes.

Procedure: Water should be filled in the tub to a level of sixteen to eighteen inches. The feet, previously warmed, should now be immersed in the tub. Friction should be continuously applied to the feet during the bath, either by an attendant or by the patient himself, by rubbing one foot against the other.

Uses: Short, cold foot bath (one to two minutes) relieves cerebral congestion and uterine haemorrhage (especially, excess bleeding during menstrual periods). When it is prolonged, it relieves sprains, strain, inflammed bunions, etc. It is also useful as diuretic measure.

Contraindication: In inflammatory conditions of the genito-urinary organs, liver and kidneys.

Hot Foot Bath

Requisites: A small tub or bucket, cold compress, a blanket.

Water Temperature: Hot water, 40 to 45°C.

Duration: Fifteen minutes.

Procedure: The patient should drink one or two glasses of cold water. The head should be protected with a cold compress. The legs, upto the calf, should be immersed in water and the patient be covered with a blanket (so that heat is not lost). During the period of treatment, the patient may be given water to drink if he feels thirsty. Immediately after the bath, he should take a cold shower.

Uses: Hot foot bath is useful to stimulate the involuntary muscles of the uterus, intestines, bladder and other pelvic and abdominal organs. It increases supply of blood to the uterus and ovaries and helps to restore delayed menstruation. This bath relieves sprains and ankle-joint pain, headache caused by cerebral congestion and cold due to chilled feet. It is also used in cases of Cold, Cough and Asthma.

Contraindication: It should be avoided in cases of high blood pressure, weakness and heart diseases.

Arm Bath

Requisites: The equipment consists of a big washbasin covered with a lid, having two opening for inserting the arms. Hot and cold water connections and a thermometer are also provided.

Water Temperature: 40 to 45°C.

Duration: Fifteen minutes.

Procedure: The patient should drink one or two glasses of cold water first, and then the arms, upto the middle of the biceps, are immersed in water. The trunk of the patient should be covered with a shawl or a blanket. Gradually, the temperature of water is raised from 40 to 45°C. At the end of the bath, hot water should be fully drained and the cold water taps opened so that the hands get a dash of cold water for a minute. Keep the limbs warm soon after drying.

Uses: The blood vessels of the hands are dilated in this bath, which facilitates draining of blood from the thoracic organs to the arms, thus relieving their congestion. This also induces perspiration, and both these reactions help to relieve Cough and any other problems connected with lungs. This treatment gives immense relief when given during an Asthma attack. It provides immediate relief in case of pain in the chest muscles.

Contraindication: As in the case of hot foot bath.

Hot Foot and Arm Bath Combined
Better results can be obtained by combining hot foot bath and arm bath for all types of headaches, broncho-nasal congestions, such

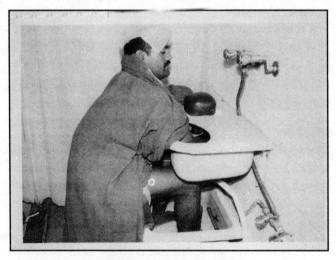

Hot Foot and Arm Bath

23

as Asthma, Cold, Sinusitis and other problems. The duration is fifteen minutes. In this bath, the temperature should gradually be increased from 40 to 45°C. The patient should be covered with a shawl or blanket around his trunk. Just as in other hot treatments, the patient should be given cold water to drink before the treatment and the head should be protected with a wet towel. A short, cold shower is to be given soon after the treatment.

Contrast Arm Bath

Requisites: For this purpose, a specially-designed tub with two compartments—one for each hand—is required, in which the water springs out as fine columns of jets, through the perforated tubes. The tubes are arranged in such a manner that the water columns cover the hands fully.

Water Temperature: Hot, 40 to 45°C, cold, 18 to 20°C.

Procedure: The patient sits on a stool and keeps both hands separately in each chamber. The tub is, then, covered with a metal sheet. First, hot water ejects through the tubes for three minutes and then cold water for one minute. This procedure is repeated four to five times, ending with cold water.

Precaution: Care should be taken that water does not fall on other parts of the body, as this interferes with blood circulation.

Uses: It gives a gentle massage to the hands, relieves congestion in other parts of the body, and various sprains and spasms. It is also helpful in treating muscular weakness and Rheumatoid Arthritis.

Contrast Foot Bath

Requisites: A specially-designed apparatus, similar to the one used in contrast arm bath, is used for this.

Water Temperature: Hot, 40 to 45°C, cold, 18 to 20°C.

Here, the water is ejected as fine columns on both legs.

Procedure and precautions: The hot and cold water treatment is the same as in contrast arm bath, just that now both legs are placed in the tub.

Uses: This gives a gentle massage to the legs and is an effective aid for relaxation. It is useful in treating Arthritis, Varicose Veins, muscular sprains and strain, and headache.

STEAM INHALATION

Requisites: Equipment used for facial sauna is very convenient for this. If this is not available, water can be heated in a vessel till steam is generated.

Duration: Five to eight minutes.

Procedure: Keep the equipment on a stool, add a cup of water and switch it on. In a little while, steam will be generated. Sit on a stool in front of the equipment, then bend over it and inhale the steam through nose and mouth by covering the head with a Turkish towel. Care should be taken not to inhale too much steam as it destroys the sensitivity of the nose and irritates the eyes. Wash the face gently with cold water and dry.

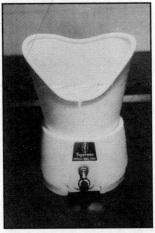

Steam Inhalation Equipment

Uses: It is useful in treating Cough, Cold, Diphtheria, Tonsillitis and Sinusitis. In acute inflammation of the pharynx, larynx and in case where the Eustachian tube is blocked due to cold, steam inhalation gives tremendous and immediate relief. It also helps in relieving headaches caused due to Sinusitis, congestion or chronic Cold. In Asthma and Emphysema cases, this acts as a powerful expectorant.

STEAM BATH

Requisites: A room specially made for this purpose. The steam is passed into the room through perforated tubes.

Duration: Ten to twelve minutes or until profuse perspiration takes place.

Procedure: The patient should drink one or two glasses of water and take a cold shower before entering the steam room. Immediately after the steam bath, a quick, cold shower is taken. A glass of cold lemon juce soon after this cold shower acts as a refresher. The patient should, then, relax for thirty to forty-five minutes.

Precautions: Sometimes, during the bath, one may feel giddy or uneasy. In such cases, the patient should immediately be taken out and cold water given to drink until the unpleasant symptoms disappear.

Uses: Steam bath is a powerful treatment to eliminate any morbid matter from the surface of the skin, a condition sometimes known as "constipation of the skin". It helps in treating cases of Arthritis (Osteo and Rheumatoid), Gout, uric acid problem and Obesity. Steam bath is helpful in all forms of chronic toxaemias. It also relieves neuralgias, such as Sciatica, facial and spinal neuralgias, functional disorders of the spinal cord, etc. It is also recommended in cases of chronic Nephritis, Migraine, malarial neuralgia, etc.

Contraindication: This bath should not be given to very weak or cardiac patients, or those suffering from high blood pressure and fever.

SAUNA BATH

Sauna bath chambers are improved replacements of the old-time Turkish bath chambers. A cabin, specially made with pine wood, is used for this purpose. Depending on the size of the cabin, two to ten patients could be treated at a time.

Duration: Twenty minutes.

Procedure: Before entering the chamber, the patient should drink plenty of cold water and take a cold shower. While in the cabin, the person should frequently rub himself to encourage dilation of the surface vessels. When he feels sufficiently hot, he should take a cold shower and return to the cabin. Finally, after inducing perspiration for the second time, the patient should take a cold shower and quickly dry himself. This should be followed by relaxation for thirty to forty minutes. A glass of cold, lemon juice will be refreshing.

Precautions: The treatment should be stopped if the patient feels giddy and should be given a cold shower immediately. Rest for twenty to thirty minutes will relieve the unpleasant symptoms.

Uses: This bath is useful in treating a majority of chronic disorders, such as Rheumatism, toxaemia of chronic Dyspepsia and Biliousness, Obesity, Sciatica, Lumbago, and all painful affliction involving large nerve trunks.

Contraindication: It is contraindicated in all cardiac diseases, eruptive skin disorders, Diabetes with emaciation, Exophthalmia, Goitre, Arteriosclerosis, Hypertension, advanced cases of Nephritis, in fever and in weakness.

SPONGE BATH

Sponge bath is given to bedridden patients who are very weak, suffering from prolonged fever/illness.

Requisites: A bucket, a Turkish towel or gloves made of Turkish cloth, a rubber sheet to cover the bed.

Duration: Three to five seconds for each part of the body.

Procedure: The patient should be covered with a bed-sheet. The towel/gloves are frequently dipped in water and the body parts are gently rubbed in this order: legs, hands, chest and abdomen. The patient is, then, turned to the other side and his back is sponged. The face and the head should be washed and dried quickly. The patient should finally be covered with a sheet.

The temperature of water depends on the effect sought and the condition of the patient. In cases of high fever, cold sponge (18 to 24°C) helps to bring down the temperature. However, for very weak patients and in fever with chills (when the patient is averse to cold), warm water may be used. Frequent sponging with warm water increases the moisture of the skin and its evaporation brings down the fever.

While using this bath for getting tonic effects, the temperature of the bath should be about 10°C and the patient should be rubbed vigorously for a duration of not more than five minutes. Cold sponge is helpful for patients suffering from Myxoedema, Cardiac and Renal Dropsy.

In hot sponging, the temperature should be as high as bearable and applied for a short duration. It helps in severe cold associated with body pain and fever, in spinal irritation, headache, Urticaria, pruritis and sleeplessness.

Alternate hot and cold sponging of the spine excites the cardiac and respiratory centres, and hence, is useful in treating all cases of toxaemia. In nervous headaches, it relaxes the central nervous system and relieves pain. It also helps in treating sprains, bruises and Rheumatoid Arthritis.

Chapter III

Jet Spray Massages

JET SPRAY MASSAGE

A jet is technically known as douche. It consists of a single, movable column of water directed under pressure against the body. In jet baths, water is employed at all temperatures for therapeutic purpose. The pressure varies from five to fifty pounds.

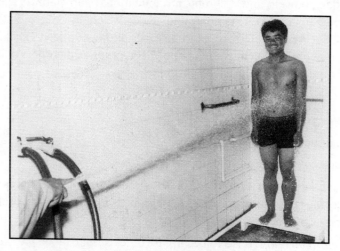

Jet Spray Massage

Cold Jet Spray Massage

Water Temperature: 18 to 24°C.

Duration: Ten seconds to three minutes.

Procedure: The patient is advised to drink a glass of cold water before the treatment and wear the abdominal guard. From a distance of five to six feet, the jet spray is directed at the back of the body first, starting from the feet and working upwards. After that, the front of the body is treated. Care is to be taken while application is made to the chest. Arms are crossed over each other and hands placed on the shoulders so that the heart and lungs are protected. No application is made to the face.

Uses: The cold jet bath is useful in treating hyperaesthesia of the skin, relieves pain in muscles and joints in chronic Rheumatism, stimulates digestion when applied to the stomach, improves circulation and assimilation and, thus, helps in cases of Anaemia. It relieves chronic indigestion with Dyspepsia, Insomnia and cerebral congestion. It stimulates nervous and muscular systems and is, therefore, helpful in treating Paralysis.

Contraindications: Cold jet bath should be avoided when there is active inflammation in the uterus, ovaries, kidneys, stomach, liver, bladder, bowels, and in chronic inflammations of all kinds. In acute Rheumatism also, it is contraindicated. It should be avoided in cases of Arteriosclerosis, heart diseases, kidney diseases, such as acute or chronic Nephritis, Gastric Ulcer, eruptive disorders of the skin, etc.

Neutral Jet Spray Massage
Water Temperature: 32 to 36°C.

Duration: Two to three minutes.

Procedure: Same as cold jet bath.

Uses: The water temperature, with pressure applied, helps in relieving body pains and improves peripheral circulation. It is useful in cases of Obesity, Arthritis, Spondylitis, etc.

Contraindication: It is avoided in case of fever, high blood pressure, heart diseases, open skin wounds, extreme weakness, etc.

Hot Jet Spray Massage
Water Temperature: 40 to 42°C.

Duration: Thirty seconds to five minutes.

Procedure: Same as cold jet spray. The temperature of water should initially be 40°C, but gradually, raised to 42°C.

Uses: Hot jet spray is useful in relieving general or superficial pains, pruritus, Urticaria, Jaundice, Neurasthenia, exhaustion, Cold, etc. Excess exposure should be avoided as it may damage the skin.

Contraindication: Same as those for neutral jet bath.

Alternate Jet Spray Massage
Procedure: In this, the hot application is followed by a short, cold application. The duration of the hot application is one to four minutes and that of the cold application three minutes.

Uses: This form of application is helpful in dealing with Sciatica, Rheumatism, Gout, Neuralgia, Obesity, etc. It relieves acute and chronic muscle pain and stimulates stomach muscles when applied to the abdominal region. It is also useful in relieving chronic pelvic congestions, such as Metritis, ovarian congestion, inflammations of the tubes, etc. This also stimulates paralysed muscles. It relieves Lumbago, uterine and ovarian neuralgia, Gastric Ulcer and chronic backache. In cerebral congestion, the application may be made to the legs. In Asthma, it may be applied to the thighs and legs. It is an ideal treatment recommended for chronic muscular Rheumatism.

Circular Jet Spray Massage
A specially made equipment directs multiple, small but powerful, water streams from all directions on the patient. This bath gives an

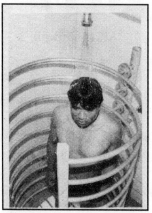

Circular Jet Spray Massage

instant cooling and refreshing effect, especially after taking a prolonged hot treatment, such as steam bath. This jet massage causes a powerful circulatory reaction, which helps in stimulating the skin's activity. It is a tonic measure for anaemics, who are fairly strong. It also stimulates muscular action. The duration is two to five minutes.

AFFUSION BATH

The affusion bath consists of single or multiple columns of water directed against a part of the body without any pressure. This was first introduced by Father Kneipp, in his Hydrotherapy Institute.

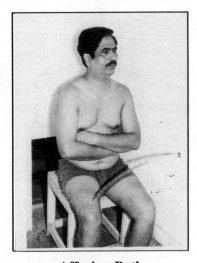

Affusion Bath

Cold Affusion

Requisites: Facility for directing cold water by means of hose pipe connected to a tap or a large mug.

Water Temperature: 18 to 24°C

Procedure: The patient comfortably sits/stands, depending on the part to be treated. Cold water is, then, poured on the specific body part.

Precaution: Care should be taken that the part is warmed before treatment.

Uses: Short (thirty seconds to three minutes) application acts as a tonic, while a longer application helps to relieve congestion. Pouring cold water on the head is helpful in reducing the temperature during fever.

Neutral Affusion

Requisites: As of cold affusion.

Water Temperature: 32 to 36°C.

Procedure: As of cold affusion.

Uses: Given to the spine, neutral affusion acts as a sedative. It also helps in relieving joint and muscular pain. Neutral affusion to the upper back acts as an expectorant and, thus, helps in cases of Asthma, Emphysema, chronic Bronchitis, respiratory tract infections, etc.

Hot Affusion

Requisites: As of cold affusion.

Water Temperature: 40 to 45°C.

Procedure: As of cold affusion. However, the hot affusion should end with a dash of cold water on the part treated.

Uses: Hot affusion helps in relieving pain in joints and muscles.

Hot and Cold Affusion

Requisites: Here, there should be two pipes to supply hot and cold water, alternately. Or else, two buckets, one with hot and the other with cold water, may be used.

Water Temperature: Hot, 42 to 45°C, cold, 18 to 20°C.

Procedure: Hot water is poured for three minutes, followed by cold for one minute. This is repeated four times, ending with cold water.

Uses: Pouring hot and cold water alternatively acts as a powerful stimulant and a tonic. It improves blood circulation to the part treated. Due to these effects, this method is employed in treating an infected part when it is impossible or undesirable to immerse the part completely in water. It relieves muscular pain and sprain. It helps to reduce pain and swelling of the joints and is, thus, helpful in Rheumatoid Arthritis.

COLD SHOWER

Many people hesitate to take cold shower thinking that they may catch cold. In fact, there is no tonic treatment better than a cold shower soon after rising every morning. It not only stimulates the blood circulation, but also activates the nerves and their centres. The person who is used to cold bath can easily continue this habit, even in the dreaded winter, without any adverse effects. The duration of the cold bath depends on the patient's condition. In case of Cold and Sinusitis patients, the bath should not be for more than two to three minutes, and while taking the bath, the person should not be exposed to cold breeze. Keep warm for some time, or if one is fit enough, moderate exercises could be done. In summer, a cold bath is very refreshing and invigorating.

Uses: The stimulating effect of the cold bath relieves one from drowsiness (due to delayed sleep), mental and physical fatigue, and helps to overcome bad habits such as alcoholism, drug addiction and smoking. Immediately after a hot treatment, a cold shower is advised to absorb the extra heat which the body acquires during the process of treatment.

This will also help to continue the reaction of the treatment. Cold shower is contraindicated in case of very weak patients, cardiac ailments, and in persons suffering from severe Cold, Influenza and Asthma.

TROMA

Requisites: Shower attached to a pipe (a hand shower).

Water Temperature: 18 to 24°C, tap water.

Duration: Ten minutes.

Procedure: A fine jet of water with moderate pressure is applied to the scalp by circular movement of the shower. It is followed by a cold pack to the head for forty-five to sixty minutes.

Uses: The gentle massage of the water columns over the scalp helps to improve circulation. Though, initially, constriction of blood vessels follows as action, later on, dilation of blood vessels takes place as reaction. In cases of Insomnia, Hypertension, Migraine,

Epilepsy, acute fever, Sun Stroke, nosebleeding, falling hair, giddiness, etc., this treatment yields remarkable results.

Contraindication: In extreme weakness, during Malarial Fever, acute Sinusitis and Asthma.

Chapter IV

Immersion Baths

IMMERSION BATH

An immersion bath is also known as full bath. It is administered in a bathtub made of porcelain or enamelled iron or fibre glass. The tub should be properly fitted with hot and cold water connections to administer the bath at cold, neutral, hot, graduated and alternate temperatures.

Cold Immersion Bath

Water Temperature: 18 to 24°C.

Duration: Fifteen minutes.

Procedure: Before entering the bathtub, the patient's head, neck and chest should be made wet with cold water and the head should be protected, preferably with a cold, moist towel (compress). The patient should enter the bathtub as quickly as possible, so as to generalise the immersion. Vigorous rubbing of the body should be done by the patient himself or by the attendant, during the bath. The bath should be terminated if the patient feels chill. Soon after the bath, the patient should be given a quick dry-up and covered with a warm blanket. If the climate is favourable, he should undertake some moderate exercises, too.

Uses: The full, cold immersion bath is advantageously employed as a routine hygienic measure. This bath is helpful in reducing high temperature during fever. It is prescribed in cases of Obesity and in Dyspepsia, to improve the appetite. This bath also improves the skin by increasing blood circulation and stimulating the activities of nerve endings. When used for this purpose, the bath should be of short duration—three to fifteen seconds.

Contraindication: This bath should not be given to young children and very old persons. It should not be given in febrile conditions caused due to acute inflammation, as in acute Peritonitis, Gastritis, Enteritis, Endometritis, Oophoritis, etc., and in cases of fever with chills.

The cold bath is contraindicated in Haematuria (blood in urine), because this condition indicates a disease either in the bladder or kidneys. (In such conditions, a short hot bath, followed by cold friction, wet sheet rubbing and a cold compress should be repeated a number of times). It should be avoided in cases of Asthma and Sinusitis.

Cold Immersion Bath with Friction
Water Temperature: 18 to 24°C.

Duration: Two to five minutes.

Procedure: The patient should quickly enter the tub and lie down. The attendant should massage the body with a Turkish towel or Turkish gloves, starting from the legs, upwards. The massage should be continued for two to five minutes or until the skin turns red. Then, the patient should take a quick shower for thirty seconds, washing the head at the same time. Thereafter, he should dry himself quickly and wear a blanket. Hyperaemia of the skin continues for fifteen to thirty minutes. Until this reaction is completed, the patient should not expose his body to cold water or cold breeze.

Uses: This treatment is helpful in reducing high temperature during fever. When a person is exposed to excess heat or sun, he should be given this bath twice or thrice to reduce the excess heat absorbed by the body. This bath is a valuable remedy for bringing down the blood pressure in hypertensives. As this bath is a powerful stimulant of the skin, it could be prescribed for all types of skin diseases like Psoriasis, where there is no inflammation of the skin. Since its effect is tonic in nature, it is useful in treating nervous and muscular disorders, including Paralysis, muscular degeneration, etc.

Contraindication: This is contraindicated for very weak patients, cardiac patients and patients suffering from kidney disorders.

Neutral Immersion Bath
Water Temperature: 32 to 36°C.

Duration: Ten to fifteen minutes. This bath can be given for a longer duration, as the water temperature is close to the body temperature. When this bath is applied for relieving Insomnia, the duration should be fifteen minutes to one hour. For Fever, it should be administered at 26 to 28°C.

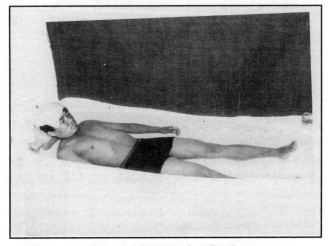

Neutral Immersion Bath

Procedure: The patient should drink one or two glasses of water before the treatment and lie in the tub after applying a cold compress to the head. After the bath, he should dry himself quickly.

Uses: It is the best sedative among all treatments. Since the neutral bath excites activity of both the skin and the kidneys, it is recommended for diseases relating to these organs. In addition, it is helpful in cases of organic diseases of the brain and spinal cord, including Paraplegia, Locomotor Ataxia, chronic inflammation of the brain and the spinal cord (such a Meningitis), Rheumatism, Arthritis and other chronic conditions.

When the neutral bath is continued at 30 to 32°C for thirty to sixty minutes or even longer, it renders great service in general Dropsy, caused due to cardiac or renal disease, where more vigorous treatments are contraindicated.

Neutral bath is also helpful for Multiple Neuritis, alcoholism and other narcotic habits, Neurasthenia, chronic Diarrhoea, Peritonitis and chronic afflictions of the abdomen, where either hot or cold water is contraindicated. In such cases, this bath may be given daily, for fifteen to thirty minutes. It is also useful in pruritus without eruption, with or without Jaundice, and in toxic conditions caused due to Dypepsia.

Contraindication: The neutral bath should not be prescribed in conditions of Eczema and other skin diseases, where water aggravates the symptoms. It is also contraindicated in extreme cardiac weakness and certain cases of Neurasthenia.

Hot Immersion Bath

Water Temperature: 40 to 42°C (above 42°C, the bath is termed as very hot).

Duration: The duration of hot bath varies from two to ten minutes, according to the temperature and condition of the patient. It should not be prolonged beyond this, as raising the heat may cause rapid congestion.

Procedure: Generally, this bath is started at 37°C and the temperature is gradually raised to the required level by adding hot water. Before entering the bath, the patient should drink sufficient quantity of cold water and wet his head, neck and shoulders with cold water. A cold compress should be applied to the head throughout the treatment.

Uses: At 40 to 44°C, for ten minutes, followed by a dry pack, it is the most efficient sweating device. This bath also relieves Capillary Bronchitis and Bronchial Pneumonia in children. At 40 to 42°C, for five to fifteen minutes, it relieves congestion of the lungs and activates the blood vessels of the skin and the muscles. As soon as the skin turns red, the bath should be terminated.

In Pneumonia and suppressed menstruation, the bath should be administered at 37.7 to 40°C, and duration be set from thirty to forty-five minutes. The bath should be given when the menstruation is due and may be repeated for two to three days in succession. For treating Dysmenorrhoea, this bath should be given at 38 to 44.4°C, for fifteen minutes.

In chronic Bronchitis, a very hot bath with friction, for five to seven minutes, should be given. This relieves congestion of the mucous membrane and gives relief immediately. After the bath, the patient should be gradually cooled and, if necessary, oil should be applied to the skin.

The hot bath at 38.8 to 41°C is a valuable treatment in chronic Rheumatism and Obesity. It can be administered for ten to fifteen minutes daily. Hot bath, taken daily, relieves the intolerable itching caused due to Jaundice and in Urticaria. When there is pain due to the formation of stone in the gall bladder or the kidneys, hot bath gives relief immediately. The pain in Cystitis is relieved by a very hot bath for ten minutes.

Contraindication: The hot bath is contraindicated in organic diseases of the brain or spinal cord, such as Tabes, Sclerosis and Myelitis. This should not be administered in cases of high blood pressure and heart diseases.

Neutral Half Bath
This bath can be conveniently taken in an immersion bathtub.

Water Temperature: 32 to 36°C.

Duration: Fifteen minutes.

Procedure: The tub is filled with water upto a height of six to eight inches. The patient should drink one or two glasses of cold water and apply cold compress over the head. Then, he should sit in the tub by stretching out his legs in the water, but keeping his arms and hands away from the water, on the sides of the tub.

Uses: When employed in case of high blood pressure, a cold compress to the chest is advised. This bath helps to relax the heart muscles and blood circulation is diverted to the lower extremities.

It also gives a soothing effect to the heart, lungs and cerebral vessels, by acting on the reflex zones present in the feet. This bath is useful in cases of Hypertension, Varicose Veins, leg cramps, Insomnia, Bronchial Asthma, Arthritis of lower limbs, Lumbago, etc.

Graduated Immersion Bath with Epsom Salt

Water Temperature: 40°C.

Duration: About thirty minutes.

Procedure: The immersion bathtub should be filled upto four to six inches of water and a pound of Epsom salt is dissolved in it. After drinking a glass of cold water and covering the head with a cold compress, the patient lies down in the tub. The attendant gives him a quick massage, starting from the legs, upwards, for two minutes. Then, the hot water tap is opened and the water level is raised to eight to ten inches at 40°C. Another pound of Epsom salt is dissolved in this water. The patient is given a massage again, for 3 to 5 minutes, starting from the legs. The patient relaxes in the tub while the cold water tap is opened, which cools the water gradually. When the tub gets filled with water, the temperature will be around 30°C and the patient should continue to relax in it for ten to twenty minutes. On coming out of the tub, he should dry himself quickly.

Uses: This bath is helpful in treatment of all types of arthritic conditions, when not associated with fever. It is also helpful as a diuretic and, hence, is useful to patients suffering from kidney disorders, Dropsy, Oedema, etc. Since this bath relaxes the whole system, it is very useful in Insomnia, too.

Contraindication: To be avoided in high blood pressure, heart diseases, weakness, Fever, etc.

ASTHMA BATH

The patient should lie down in the immersion tub, which is half filled with water, at a temperature of 37 to 38°C. The hot water tap is then opened and temperature raised upto 40 to 42°C. The duration is four minutes. Then, the body is rubbed, beginning with the left leg, then the left arm, abdomen, chest, right arm, right leg, back and the spine. The spine is rubbed till the skin turns red. After rubbing the spine, the chest and the abdomen are rubbed again, for three to four minutes. When rubbing is over, the flow of hot water is stopped. Then, the patient is asked to sit in an upright position and exhale for an instant, and a bucketful of cold water is splashed over his back. Immediately, the patient is asked to inhale and half a bucket of cold water is poured on his chest. He is asked to lie in the tub again for two to four minutes.

This process has to be repeated twice or thrice. The water in the tub has to be brought back always to 37 to 38°C. Finally, a short, cold shower for two minutes, and thirty to forty minutes of relaxation is advised.

Uses: This treatment helps to improve the depth of respiration and relieves congestion from the lungs. Hence, it is helpful in Asthma, Bronchitis, Emphysema, etc.

WHIRLPOOL BATH

Water Temperature: Cold, 18 to 24°C, neutral, 32 to 36°C.

Duration: Fifteen minutes.

Procedure: The water revolves in a big well-type tub. When the patient enters the tub, he gets a gentle massage by the whirling water. A normal adult can take this bath with cold water.

Uses: This bath is a powerful stimulant for muscular and circulatory activities. When given with cold water, it reduces the temperature of the body, but stimulates perspiration, heart's activity and other vital functions. Since the cold bath increases the blood pressure, it is not advisable for high blood pressure patients. Due to the increased respiratory movement there will be rigorous fluxion through the brain, thereby making the brain more alert and active. The sudden contact of cold water stimulates the activity of the kidneys, liver and peristalsis of the intestines; hence, it is useful in chronic Constipation and disorders of the kidney and liver. Persons emaciated due to deficient absorption of nutrition will benefit, as this increases the appetite as well as the digestion and assimilation of food. It may be given after giving hot applications like steam bath, sun bath, sauna bath, etc., for a short duration.

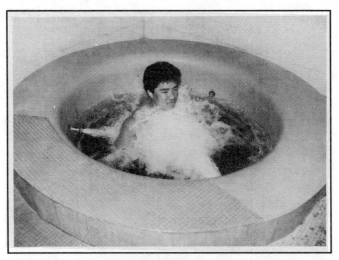

Whirlpool Bath

Like other neutral baths, the neutral whirlpool bath is also relaxing and causes passive dilation of the peripheral blood vessels. The impact made upon the muscular tissues is profound and the tissue toxins are quickly excreted during this treatment. This bath is useful in all irritable conditions of the brain, nervous and muscular systems.

UNDERWATER PRESSURE MASSAGE

This is the latest addition to hydrotherapeutics. By this application, the body gets influenced not only with the temperature of the water, but also by the percussion movement, which is made on the periphery with a strong water jet. In fact, this is the combination of two treatments, viz., general immersion bath and massage.

Cold Underwater Massage

Water Temperature: Cold, 18 to 24°C, or neutral, 32 to 36°C.

Duration: Fifteen minutes.

Procedure: This treatment is given in a specially fabricated tub with an attached jet pipe. In case of neutral underwater massage, the patient must drink one or two glasses of cold water before the treatment. He is subjected to a gentle vibration of the water, and later, a jet spray is directed over his back and front.

A short, cold shower is given to the head after the neutral underwater massage and the patient is advised to relax for thirty to forty minutes.

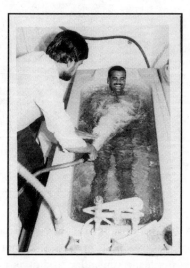

Underwater Pressure Massage

Uses: Cold underwater massage is helpful in stimulating the activity of the skin by diversion of circulation to the peripheral blood vessels. The muscles absorb the excess heat and tone up. Hence, it is useful in strengthening muscles, whenever there is atony.

In cases of Paralysis, Poliomyelitis and Paraplegia, cold underwater massage is a valuable treatment. It not only stimulates the activity of the skin, but also the entire nervous system (because of its strong reaction on the nerve ends). Hence, this is useful in all types of neuralgias. And since the cold underwater massage stimulates the digestive activity and increases the production of gastric juices, it is useful for patients suffering from loss of appetite due to deficient secretion of these digestive juices.

Neutral Underwater Massage
The neutral underwater massage at 32 to 36°C is a relaxing treatment, especially after a rigorous physical activity, such as exercising, walking, etc. After participation in sports and games,

this treatment relaxes the tired muscles. It is a also useful in cases of Insomnia and helps to tone up muscular and nervous systems. In cases of Spondylosis, Sciatica, Arthritis, Scoliosis and other disorders of the bones and joints, neutral underwater massage proves useful.

Chapter V

Enema

ENEMA

Enema is an injection of fluid into the rectum. It is also known as rectal irrigation.

Requisites: An enema can.

Water Temperature: Lukewarm.

Procedure: The patient lies down on his right, extending his right leg and folding the left leg at a right angle. The enema nozzle, which is smeared with oil or vaseline, is introduced into the rectum. Slowly, the can is raised to a height of three feet from the patient and water is allowed to enter the rectum. If the patient feels pain during this process, the height of the can should be reduced and the flow of water stopped for a while. The pain will then subside. The enema can is again raised to three feet. Generally, two to four pints of water is injected into the rectum. Great care should be taken to avoid entry of air into the bowels, as this may cause severe colic pain. When there is pain due to gases while giving enema, a gentle massage over the colon region will relieve the same. Large quantities of water should not be injected, as this may sometimes cause damage by distending the colon. The water has to be retained for at least five to ten minutes. The patient should take a short walk while retaining the water and then go to the toilet, where he should slowly expel the water along with accumulated morbid matter. The patient should not hasten to release all the water at once.

Uses: Warm water enema is helpful in cleaning the rectum of the accumulated faecal matter. This is the safest method known to the medical world for cleaning the bowels. This also improves the peristaltic movements of the bowels and, thereby, relieves Constipation. Cold enema, at 18°C, is helpful in inflammatory conditions of the colon, especially in Dysentery, Diarrhoea, ulcerative Colitis, Haemorrhoids and in Fever. Hot enema, at 40 to 42°C, is helpful in relieving irritation due to inflammatory pain of the rectum and pain of Haemorrhoids. It is also helpful in Dysmenorrhoea and Leucorrhoea. In some cases, where there is an infection in the colon, such as Amoebiasis, infective Colitis or worm infestation, enema may be administered with neem water (a decoction prepared by boiling neem leaves in water).

Graduated Enema
This procedure is adopted to discontinue the habit of taking regular enema. On the first day, the person is given enema with three pints of water at body temperature. On the succeeding days, the amount of water is reduced by half pint per day. During the last three days, the person may be given enema with half a pint of water, just to stimulate the activity of the rectum.

VAGINAL IRRIGATION
It is commonly known as vaginal douche. Here, water is introduced into the vaginal canal, with very little or no pressure.

Requisites: For giving this application, a special type of nozzle is used. This nozzle may be attached to an enema can or to a tube connected to a rubber bag.

Water Temperature: Cold, neutral or hot.

Procedure: The patient lies on the back with her hips slightly elevated. A proper receptacle is placed to collect the water as it flows out from the vagina. Care should be taken to introduce the nozzle at the back of the uterus. The water circulates through the vagina, bringing all the parts of it under the thermic influence of the application.

The reaction occurs not only in the mucous membrane of the vagina, but also reflexively influences circulation in the pelvic organs.

I) Cold Irrigation

It is useful in Menorrhagia, especially when there is inflammation in the genital organs. When the cold application is continued for ten to fifteen minutes, it stimulates uterine activity. The cold irrigation is helpful in Burning Micturation and in reducing irritability of the vaginal canal in case of urinary tract infections.

II) Neutral Irrigation

It is said to relax the irritability of the vaginal canal and uterus in conditions like Leucorrhoea and vaginal pruritus, especially in diabetics. It is proved in several cases that the application of vaginal irrigation regulates menstruation, when applied along with other treatments like hot hip bath.

III) Hot Irrigation

Uses: Hot irrigation, at 40°C, relieves pain and stimulates blood circulation in diseases like Salpingitis, Cellulitis, chronic Metritis, Oophoritis and Endometritis.

Hot irrigation must be avoided during pregnancy as it may induce miscarriage. But after the beginning of labour, it induces prompt dilation of the cervix. Alternate hot and cold vaginal irrigation is a powerful stimulant for pelvic organs.

Chapter VI

Mud Therapy

Mud is one of the five elements of nature having immense impact on the body in health, as well as in sickness. It can be employed conveniently as a therapeutic agent in naturopathy treatment as its black colour absorbs all the colours of the sun and conveys them to the body. Secondly, as the mud retains moisture for a long time, it cools the body when applied over it. Thirdly, its shape and consistency can be changed easily by adding water. Last, but not the least, it is cheap and easily available.

Mud procured for treatment purpose should be black, cotton soil with greasiness, but free from pollution and contamination. Before use, the mud should be dried, powdered and sieved to separate stones, grass particles and other impurities.

MUDPACK (LOCAL APPLICATION)

Method: It is applied by keeping water-soaked mud in a thin, wet muslin cloth and making it into a thin, flat brick, depending on the size of the patient's abdomen. The size of mudpacks are generally ten inches by six inches by one inch for adults. The duration of the mudpack application is twenty to thirty minutes. When applied in cold weather, place a blanket over the mudpack and cover the body as well.

Uses: When applied to abdomen, it relieves all forms of indigestion. It is effective in decreasing intestinal heat and stimulates peristalsis. A thick mudpack applied to head, in congestive headache, relieves the pain immediately. The advantage of mudpack over cold compress is that it retains the coolness for a longer time. Hence, it is recommended whenever there is a necessity for a prolonged cold application.

MUDPACK FOR FACE

Fine mud-paste is applied on the face and allowed to dry for thirty minutes. This is helpful in improving the complexion of the skin, removing pimples and opening skin pores, which in turn facilitate elimination of toxins. It is also helpful in removing dark circles around the eyes. After thirty minutes, the face should be washed thoroughly with cold water.

MUDPACK FOR EYES

Soaked mud, to a size of half inch thickness, is placed in a nine by six inch, wet cloth. It is then folded on all sides like the mudpack applied on the abdomen. It is placed on the eyes for twenty to thirty minutes.

Uses: It reduces irritation of the eyes and, hence, is useful in cases of Conjuctivitis, Haemorrhage in the eye ball, itching of the eyes, allergic conditions, etc. It is also useful in cases of errors of refraction like short-sightedness and long-sightedness, and is especially useful in Glaucoma, where it helps to reduce eye ball tension. It also provides relaxation to the eyes.

MUDBATH

Duration: Forty-five to sixty minutes.

Procedure: It is given in a special cubicle where the patient can expose himself to sunlight. Mud may be applied to the patient in a sitting or lying position. This helps to improve the skin condition by increasing blood circulation and energising the skin tissues. Care should be taken to avoid catching of cold during the bath. Afterwards, the patient must be thoroughly washed with cold water jet spray. It the patient feels chill, warm water should be used. The patient is, then, dried quickly and transferred to a warm bed.

Uses: Mudbath invigorates the circulatory system by diverting a large amount of blood to the periphery and, hence, is useful in cleansing and strengthening the skin tissue.

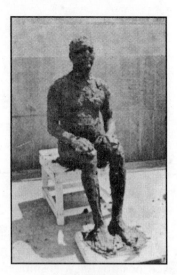

Mudbath

Taking frequent mudbath helps in improving the complexion of the skin by getting rid of spots and patches, which appear in various skin disorders, especially after chickenpox and smallpox. Mudbath is also generally recommended for all skin diseases, including Psoriasis, Leucoderma, Leprosy, Urticaria and other allergic conditions of the skin. Mud applications are a part of natural beauty treatment.

Chapter VII

Massage

OIL MASSAGE

Oil massage is a treatment in which oil is smeared all over the body and kneaded in a systematic manner. The patient is made to lie down in a relaxed position on a cushioned table, designed specially for the purpose. The massage movements are made manually by a masseur. The movements are regulated according to the part that is to be treated. Movements like percussion, friction, kneading, stroking and vibration are made for a period of thirty minutes.

The movements are effected in the direction of venous blood flow. To start with, the massage is done on the right side of the

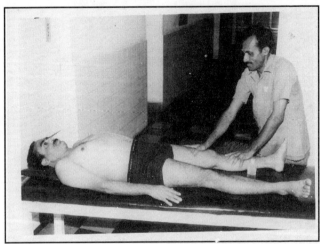

Oil Massage

body—beginning from the right foot—and then, the head and neck. After the oil massage, the patient is asked to take a sunbath for twenty minutes and, then, a warm water bath.

Uses: Massage relaxes the body. It also helps to improve blood circulation. The pressure applied over the body part, by means of various massage movements, makes the blood flow into the major vessels of venous circulation system. This increased venous circulation steps up the arterial circulation and helps in conveying nourishment and oxygen to various parts of the body.

Massage also helps in improving skin activity and its excretory function, by cleaning the skin pores and activating sweat and sebaceous glands that are embedded in the skin. The nervous system is also influenced by stimulation of the millions of nerve endings that are located in the skin.

Contraindication: Massage is avoided during fever, pregnancy, menstruation, skin eruptions, Diarrhoea, Dysentery, acute inflammation and fasting.

VIBRO-MASSAGE

In this massage, talcum power is applied as a medium and the movements are performed by a machine. For this purpose,

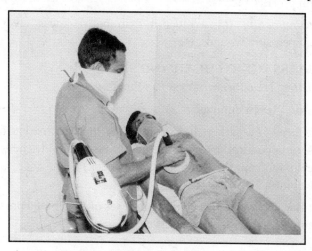

Vibro Massage

different applicators are used on different parts of the body. The immense vibration applied on any body part influences the circulatory and nervous systems. The duration of the massage is thirty minutes.

Contraindication: Vibro-massage is avoided in case of Fever, acute inflammation, menstruation, pregnancy, weakness, Diarrhoea, Dysentery and during fasting.

COLD FRICTION
Requisites: A hot water bag, a glove made of Turkish cloth, a blanket, a bucket of cold water.

Water Temperature: 18 to 22°C.

Duration: Fifteen minutes.

Procedure: The patient is made to lie face downwards on the table, with a hot water bag at his feet. The attendant dips the glove in cold water and applies brisk friction to the patient, starting from the feet and working upwards, part by part, including the front and back. Each part that has been rubbed, is covered with a blanket. A short, cold shower is given after the treatment.

Uses: This is useful in treating hypertension, fever without rigors, general pruritis, etc.

Contraindication: It is avoided in extreme weakness, fever with chills, open skin wounds, etc.

ICE MASSAGE TO HEAD AND SPINE
Requisites: Ice cubes wrapped in a thin towel.

Duration: Seven minutes.

Procedure: The patient lies prone, with the back exposed. Ice cubes, wrapped in the towel, are gently moved along the length of the spine, from the occiput (base of neck) to the coccyx (end of the spine).

Uses: It is a very useful treatment in cases of high blood pressure, as it acts on the sympathetic nerves.

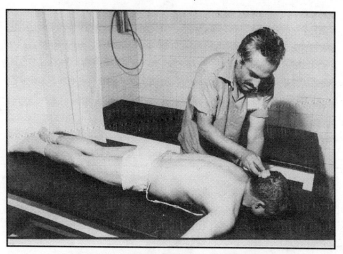

Ice Massage to Head and Spine

Migraine headaches also respond well to this application, when applied to the back of the neck and head.

Chapter VIII

Physiotherapy

SONOPULS

It is an application of ultrasound for the treatment of both superficial lesions and deep tissues.

Uses: This therapy is indicated in cases of Osteoarthritis, Tendinitis, Bursitis, Capsulitids, Spondylorthrosis and Trismus.

In this therapy, powerful short waves are produced and passed through the patient's body by heating of tissues using condensor pads. It relieves pain and stimulates splanchnic nerves. It also helps to increase the leucocytes (white blood cells) count and destroys micro-organisms.

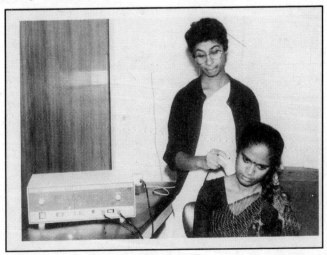

Sonopuls

Uses: Helpful in cases of neuralgia, Peripheral Nerve Paralysis, Rheumatism, Scapular Periarthritis, sprain, Osteoarthritis, Myositis, etc.

Contraindication: Avoid in cases of ulcers of the stomach, Tuberculosis, tumours in the abdominal organs and heart diseases.

ENDOMED
It helps in relieving pain and induces muscle contraction without any unpleasant sensation. It is useful in treatment of very sensitive areas (e.g., stimulation of perineal muscles in case of incontinence).

Uses: Good for treatment of Peripheral Nerve Paralysis, Progressive Muscle Dystrophy, Paralysis, muscle spasm, Capsulitis, Fibrositis, Myositis, etc.

TRANSCUTANEOUS ELECTRICAL NERVE STIMULATOR (TENS)
It is one of the best-established and the most widely used methods of electrical activation of afferent fibres, of both muscles and skin. It is very effective in alleviating pain. Relief begins after a few minutes of stimulation, which is usually experienced as a mild vibration.

It is useful in muscular spasms, acute oro-facial pain caused by periodontal infections, cervical strain, Migraine, chronic back pain, sports injuries, etc.

CERVICAL AND LUMBAR INTERMITTENT TRACTIONS
This traction unit is based on motor gear and lever system.

Uses: Helpful in treating Cervical and Lumbar Spondylosis, and degenerative changes.

MILL TRAC COMPUTER
This traction is programmed through a computer system. In this trac computer, the following tractions can be given:
- Horizontal tractions
- Intermittent static tractions
- Intermittent force tractions

These are helpful in cases of degenerative changes, and Cervical and Lumbar Spondylosis.

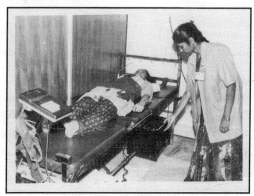

Mill Trac Computer

WAX BATH

Molten wax at 42 to 45°C, is applied to the affected areas, and allowed to cool down to body temperature in ten to fifteen minutes. Like fomentation, wax baths are also useful in treating chronic conditions like Arthritis, Arthritis Deformans and deep-seated muscle pain caused due to sprain.

MYO-MATIC

Uses: Helpful in cases of acute and chronic pains of Spondylosis, Osteoarthritis, sports injuries, etc.

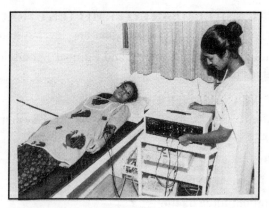

Myo-matic

VASOTRAIN

Vacuum/Compression Therapy Unit: This helps in maintaining optimum blood supply to the lower limbs, which is often restricted in diabetic patients. In case of long-standing restriction on blood circulation, the part may become gangrenous. Vasotrain helps in preventing/postponing amputation of such part.

Uses: Helps in activating the peripheral tissues in case of Diabetes, Gangrene, Hypertension, radiating pain and burning sensation in limbs.

LASER THERAPY

The word laser is an acronym for "Light Amplification by Stimulated Emission of Radiation". This definition aptly describes the operation of a laser, consisting of emitted light, which is therefore photonic and may be visible or invisible depending on its wavelength. The emission is first stimulated by an electromagnetic radiation so that the incident and induced rays coincide, resulting in a ray with strictly identical parameters (frequency, phase, energy). At its basic photonic level, the laser beam is no different from ordinary light. It is a concentrated regrouping of photons emitted in phase that produces a coherent and powerful beam. There is no such thing as laser light, rather only a laser effect applicable to the light.

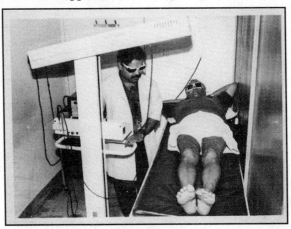

Laser Beam

59

Laser therapy is useful in decreasing both swelling and pain, and helps in fast recovery by promoting elasticity of ligaments, relaxation and bone and tissue repair. Thus, laser therapy is useful in muscle pulls, sprains, Tendinitis, muscle spasms, Tennis Elbow, swollen/twisted ankle, traumatic blows, Arthritis and Bursitis.

Chapter IX
Diet

DIET

Diet is broadly divided into three kinds:

- Eliminative Diet
- Soothing Diet
- Constructive Diet

According to naturopathy, the root cause of most of the diseases is the accumulation of morbid matter in the digestive system. It is essential to cleanse it by diverting the energies of the body by fasting. Fasting is essential in almost all diseases. Ayurveda states that it helps not only in cleaning the digestive system, but also all the seven ingredients of the body (lymph, blood, muscle, cartilage, bone marrow, bone and sperm). Fasting is not recommended for very weak patients, pregnant women, person of advanced age, infants and TB patients. During the fasting period, the patients may be put on water, lime juice or fresh juice, depending on their general vitality and seriousness of the disease. The patients should also be given regular enema, cold towel packs, bath, rest and relaxation. Fasting results in some difficulty during the first two days, but, later, one can fast for as long as he starts feeling hungry again. During fasting, the following symptoms may occur: tastelessness, bad odour from the mouth, coated tongue, vomiting, slight pain in the stomach, giddiness, exhaustion, etc. All these symptoms appear because of the beginning of the process of elimination of morbid matter from the body. It is advisable to continue the fast until the tongue gets cleared, appetite becomes normal and the patient feels energetic again.

No patient should experiment fasting without proper guidance. It is always advisable to fast under the supervision of an expert naturopath. Meanwhile, the patient should not get involved in strenuous mental activities like business, official work and should be free from worries. Only tolerable physical activities, in the form of treatment (light yogasanas and walking), are permitted.

In soothing diet, fruit juices, gruels, butter-milk, vegetable soups, vegetable juices, raw salads, boiled vegetables, wheat and rice preparations in limited quantity are recommended.

Vegetables, such as cabbage, celery, lettuce, and roots like carrot, string beans, gourds may be used in the diet. Ripe fruits of all sorts are of great value because they contain germ-destroying acids. Sometimes, patients are put on a fruit diet consisting of seasonal fruit and raw vegetables. Fruits and vegetables should be chewed properly while eating. This helps the body in digesting the sugar secreted, in the mouth itself. Intestinal asepsis may be promoted by fruits and butter-milk. If raw diet is not masticated well, it may lead to production of gases.

A full meal, which consists of curds, milk, boiled vegetables, chapatis, rice, dal, etc., is given in a constructive diet.

Meat of all kinds, tea, coffee and animal broths are strictly excluded because of the presence of tissue wastes, uric acid, creatinine and other substances, which are the products of putrefactive changes.

The diet should consist of boiled vegetables, without addition of any type of irritants. *Sattvik* diet is good for all, whether sick or not. The diet should be well-planned for treating Fever, Obesity, nutritional disorders, Indigestion, Jaundice, Hepatic Cirrhosis, all forms of auto-intoxication, Bright's disease, Malaria, Tuberculosis, Eczema, Anaemia, acute infections and inflammatory disorders of all types, and acute and chronic ailments of the body. Diets including pickles, preserved/fried food, coffee, tea, cocoa, alcohol and condiments consisting of mustard, pepper, hot sauces should be avoided.

Diseases
and
Their Treatments

In the following chapters, our aim is to help the patients in implementing suitable, prescribed treatments soon after the onset of the disease so that the disease does not progress further; and the treatment acts as a first-aid in preventing any forthcoming disease. This part of the book emphasises the treatment to be taken in a particular disease, with its therapeutic use in frequency, and hence will serve as a ready reckoner for most of the common ailments and their treatment. However, it is always wise to refer the patients to a naturopath rather than experimenting with one or the other treatment, particularly when the situation seems to be out of control. The treatments mentioned here are more preventive and harmless in nature, and have no side effects if implemented with necessary precautions and guidelines. We hope our readers will understand the limits and follow the same as and when these treatments are required.

Chapter X

Nutrition and Metabolic Disorders

OBESITY

Obesity is a complex disorder of the modern world. It is defined as an abnormal increase in weight of the body—over ten per cent above the desirable level—caused due to generalised deposition of fat.

Social factors have a marked bearing on the prevalence of Obesity and certain situations affect greatly on the eating habits of an obese person. Negative lifestyle habits, which contribute to Obesity, include:

- Improper dietary habits
- Lack of physical exercise/entertaining sedentary habits
- Intake of alcohol, excessive tea, coffee, *paan*, *zarda*, smoking, etc.
- Stress and strain

Obesity has one basic cause—intake of more food than required, coupled with lack of exercise. Although most cases of Obesity are due to simple overeating habits, caused by emotional, familial, metabolic and genetic factors, a few cases due to endocrine disorders have also been reported.

Depending on the excess weight, Obesity can be classified as:

- Mild to Moderate   – Ten to twenty per cent above desirable weight.
- Moderate to Severe – Twenty to thirty per cent above desirable weight.

- Severe Obesity — Thirty per cent above desirable weight.

Treatment

- Cold hip bath, twice daily (if the weather is favourble). Fifteen to twenty minutes is advisable.

- Oil massage, once a week, improves general health and helps in mobilising fat.

- Steam and sauna baths increase the body's basal metabolic rate and help as an adjuvant in losing weight.

- Warm water immersion baths with Epsom salt, for fifteen to twenty minutes duration, too, are helpful.

- Friction baths, graduated immersion baths, neutral whirlpool and underwater massage are also beneficial.

- Any other treatment used for improving general health could be employed in the treatment of Obesity.

- Warm water enema, regularly for the first three to four days of fasting, and thereafter, every alternate day during extended periods of fasting, is beneficial.

- Fasting, initially, for a period of three to four days, on low calorie liquids, such as lemon juice and adequate intake of fluids, is useful.

- Fasting once a week thereafter is adequate.

- After breaking the fast, one should be mentally prepared to go on a low calorie diet, coupled with regular physical exercise, like walking at a pace of five km/hour for an hour, yoga and freehand warm-up exercises, till the desirable weight is reached. However, some exercises should be continued even after that.

DIABETES MELLITUS

High standard of living has enabled almost everyone to select and eat from a vast array of food items. In the industrially developed countries, the sheer abundance of food has proved a mixed blessing. Refrigeration and sophisticated food preserving and processing techniques have made it possible to store fatty food for a longer period of time, which otherwise would have turned rancid within a short duration, if kept unused. In addition, lack of physical exercise due to sedentary habits, coupled with stressful living, has led to greater health hazards such as Obesity, Diabetes, coronary heart ailments, kidney diseases, neck and back pains, etc.

Surveys done in the field, for the last twenty-five years, show that the incidence of Diabetes Mellitus has increased by three to four per cent, both in developed as well as in developing countries. Urbanites appear to be more prone to Diabetes than the rural people.

Diabetes is a condition where the blood sugar level increases. It is broadly classified as Insulin-Dependent or Juvenile Diabetes, (where insulin should be given to control blood sugar) and Non-Insulin Dependent Diabetes, which can be controlled by diet and exercises alone.

There are several factors which pre-dispose a person to Diabetes, such as strong family history of Diabetes Mellitus, Obesity, physical inactivity, stress, trauma and overeating. General symptoms of Diabetes are excessive thirst, hunger and urination. Weight loss and weakness may also be seen.

Treatment
- Mudpacks over the abdomen, daily, for fifteen to twenty minutes, improve blood circulation to abdominal and pelvic region, enhancing their functional capacity, specially of liver and pancreas. Cold towel pack can also be used instead of mudpacks.
- Cold hip baths, for fifteen to twenty minutes daily, if the weather is conducive, also yield the above benefits.
- Warm water enema, regularly in the morning, for two to three days, helps in clearing accumulated wastes from the large intestine.
- Warm water immersion baths and cold friction baths, for a period of twenty and ten minutes, respectively, are also beneficial.
- Body massage, once a while, improves blood circulation, tones up the muscles and improves general health.

- Abdominal pack, applied at night, three hours after meal, activates abdominal organs, especially liver and pancreas. It also helps inducing good digestion and enhances the metabolic rate.

- Steam and sauna baths, generally, raise basal metabolic rate and burn up excessive calories by breaking down the carbohydrates. They also help in proper peripheral utilisation of glucose.

- Alternate hip baths—three minutes hot and one minutes cold, four to five times, ending with cold hip bath, help to stimulate digestive organs. They can be taken twice a week.

- Gastro-hepatic pack is also useful in Diabetes and other gastro-intestinal problems. It should be taken twice or thrice a week.

- Mudbath improves blood circulation to skin, diverting a large amount of blood to periphery, thus improving skin function, which is usually poor in diabetic patients.

- Regular exercise, such as walking, yogasanas, pranayama and yoganidra, should form an important aspect of the treatment.

Many of the Non-Insulin Dependent Diabetes do not require drugs to control blood sugar levels. Regulated diet and regular physical exercise is all that he is required to do to control blood sugar levels.

Though the diet of a diabetic is in no way different from the diet of a normal individual, the following aspects should be kept in mind:

- Daily intake of calories must be reduced by those who are overweight.

- Fat intake should be restricted, especially oils rich in monosaturated and saturated fatty acids (e.g. ghee, vanaspati, butter, etc.).

- Intake of food should be restricted to small, frequent meals. Skipping meal in between, prolonged fasting or fasting without guidance from a professional should be avoided.

- Fibre-rich foods should be included in the diet.
- Complex carbohydrates to be preferred to simple sugars (e.g., carbohydrates derived from cereals, grains and legumes).
- The diet of a diabetic should consist of sixty to seventy per cent carbohydrates, ten to fifteen per cent fats and fifteen to twenty per cent proteins.
- Sugar, honey, cakes, sherbets, fried foods, syrups, alcohol, tender coconuts, jackfruits, mangoes, bananas, sapotas (chikoo) and custard apples should be totally avoided.

Chapter XI

Disorders of the Musculo- Skeletal System

Arthritis is truly an universal illness like Hypertension, Diabetes, Obesity and digestive disorders—a disease of the unhealthy lifestyle of the modern world. Prevention of Arthritis is actually better than cure, although all forms of Arthritis can be treated.

Arthritis is the inflammation of a joint. It has many types and as many as ninety-six of them have been identified. When a joint becomes arthritic, there will be swelling and damage to the underlying tissue. Pain and stiffness are the most common symptoms one experiences. As the disease progresses, the range of motion gradually diminishes, with the joint becoming increasingly stiff. Once the joint becomes stiff, the muscles around it are not exercised adequately and they shrink in size, resulting in muscular weakness, known as Disuse Atrophy. This, in turn, leads to increased risk of injury to joints and the arthritic condition aggravates. The current enthusiasm for running, aerobics and jogging, for both pleasure and fitness, also results in some musculo-skeletal problems.

HOW DOES A JOINT WORK?
Before going into the details about Arthritis, let us take a look at how a joint works. There are several types of joints in the body. Some are highly mobile, some stable and mobile, and some immobile.

What is amazing about the human body is its architectural arrangement of bones, muscles and joints, strong enough to support its weight, rigid enough to protect the soft internal organs, and flexible enough to provide the agility that ensures man's survival.

Although the joint formation varies with the type of joint, most joints are made up of the same elements. The joint is enclosed in a tough, fibrous capsule of connective tissue, which secretes the synovial fluid, a fluid which lubricates the moving parts. Outside this capsule, the fibrous anchors, called ligaments, surround the joint and link the two bones protecting the capsule and keeping the movements of the joint within safe limit. An American novelist, Herman Melville, observed, "The human body is like a ship, its bones being the stiff rigging, and the tendons small, running ropes that manage all the motions."

WHAT CAN GO WRONG WITH A JOINT?

The simplest example is a sprain, an ankle injury caused by a twist of the foot. The joint becomes swollen with fluid, the blood supply to the part increases and it becomes warm and painful. Movements become restricted because of the swelling and pain. In a fracture of the bone, even if pain is not severe, one feels instinctively that one should avoid putting weight on it. A sprain becomes better after some time, while a fracture takes time to heal. During an attack of Gout, the joint is inflamed, whereas in Rheumatoid Arthritis, there is no such obvious reason and the disease itself appears to be the source of inflammation.

There are several kinds of Arthritis:

- *Degenerative*—Osteoarthritis, Cervical and Lumbar Spondylitis.

- *Inflammatory*—Rheumatoid Arthritis, Ankylosing Spondylitis and Psoriatic Arthritis.

- *Infective*—Bacterial Pneumo, Gono, Meningo, Strepto and Styphylo, and viral (Rubella).

- *Metabolic*—Gout.

OSTEOARTHRITIS

The most frequent form of Arthritis is Osteoarthritis, a wear and tear disease that becomes increasingly common with age. It results from a wearing down of the cartilage in the joints. The pads of cartilages at the ends of the bones become splayed and rough instead of smooth, preventing normal movements of the joints. The joints begin to grate like a rusty gate, instead of operating smoothly like a well-oiled machine. Osteoarthritis mostly affects the large, weight-bearing joints—knees and hips—as well as spine.

Gravity is the main enemy of man's weight-bearing joints. The repeated impact on them causes minute trauma everytime and leads to degeneration of the joint, i.e. osteoarthritic changes set in. Naturally, people who are overweight are more likely to suffer from this.

Osteoarthritis often follows an injury to or a repeated abuse of a joint, as often in case of athletes. It is still not known why many people who subject their joints to constant abuse often escape from Osteoarthritis, while others suffer from it.

Pain and stiffness are the most common symptoms, which are usually noticed with weather changes. Sometimes, the affected joints become tender and swollen.

Treatment

The frequency and the duration of the treatment varies depending on its severity and the effect sought.

Osteoarthritis of the Knee and Ankle Joints

The following treatments are useful in relieving pain and swelling of the knee and ankle joints.

- Gentle massage to the joints to strengthen muscles around them.
- Hot and cold fomentation and affusion to the joints to relieve pain and spasm.
- Cold compresses to joints to treat localised inflammation and pain.
- A heating compress is also helpful in relieving pain/stiffness/ swelling.

- Neutral immersion and neutral half bath with Epsom salt, for fifteen to twenty minutes.
- Contrast foot baths are also very helpful in relieving pain and spasm.
- Neutral jet, whirlpool and underwater massages help in relaxing the muscles of joints.
- Direct, hot mud applications relieve pain.
- Regular exercises, such as flexion and extension of the joints, help to strengthen the muscles.

It is also important to reduce weight by following a controlled diet programme under the guidance of a doctor.

RHEUMATOID ARTHRITIS

It is a systemic or whole body disease. In addition to stiff, hot, painful and swollen joints, many patients experience acute fatigue, weakness, fever, malaise, loss of appetite, Anaemia and weight loss. Connective tissue and organs in the body, including heart, lungs, nerves and eyes, may get damaged.

Again, as in many other diseases, the exact cause of Rheumatoid Arthritis is not known. It is an autoimmune disorder in which the body attacks its own tissues. There is often hereditary predisposition, though the disease is not inherited.

Damage to the joints results from the inflammation of the synovial membrane, which produces the fluid to lubricate the joints. Prolonged inflammation destroys the cartilage and weakens the ligaments of the joint. It may even damage the tendons. Muscles attached to the inflamed joint become weak and painful due to spasm. These spasms restrict movement of the muscle and lead to further weakness—a condition known as Disuse Atrophy. When Rheumatoid Arthritis progresses further, deformities set in and cripple the person.

Joints most commonly affected are the proximal smaller joints, fingers, base of toes, wrists, knees, ankles, shoulders, hips and elbows.

Women are three times more susceptible than men to Rheumatoid Arthritis.

Treatment

- If detected and treated early, many Rheumatoid Arthritis sufferers can lead a normal life without being crippled.
- Regular, physical exercises with strict adherence to diet, avoiding milk and milk products. A common misconception among many people is that lime juice is not good for Arthritis. But it is not true. In fact, lime juice, which has Vitamin C, helps in strengthening the connective tissue that binds the bones.
- Frequent warm water baths.
- Neutral immersion and neutral half bath for upto twenty minutes duration.
- Steam and sauna bath once in a while.
- Hot/cold affusion or fomentation to the affected joints.
- Periodic hot foot and arm bath.
- Cold pack to the inflammed joints daily.
- Hot mud application to the affected joints.
- Infrared ray treatment, followed by direct mud application, to the affected joint.
- Warm water jet massage, underwater massage and whirlpool baths are also useful.

GOUTY ARTHRITIS

Gout is a metabolic disease and often runs in families. It is associated with abnormal accumulation of urates in the body and is characterised early by a recurring acute Arthritis, usually mono-articular (single joint involvement), and later on, deforming chronic Arthritis. About ninety per cent of patients of Gout are men, usually of over thirty years of age.

In acute Gouty Arthritis, involvement of peripheral joint, mainly metatarsal joint of the big toe, is common. It becomes so much red, hot, swollen and tender that even the soft touch of bedclothes may become agonising. The attack is insidious, sometimes explosively sudden and may even wake up the patient from sleep.

After a few days, the symptoms and signs usually disappear, followed by peeling of skin overlying the affected joint. Attacks may recur after weeks, months or even years.

In chronic Gouty Arthritis, recurrent attacks of Gout result in progressive erosion of the cartilage and bone associated with the formation of tophi (urate crystal deposition), causing considerable disability with Osteoarthritis superimposed over it. Tophi are nodular thickenings which occur in tendon sheaths, bursae and cartilage of the ear. Renal Caliculi (stones in the kidneys) occur in about ten per cent of Gout sufferers. The uric acid level in the blood would, then, be high.

Treatment

Treatment used for Osteoarthritis of knees and ankles hold good for Gouty Arthritis also.

To help reduce high blood uric acid level, the following items should be avoided.

- Meat, fish and other non-vegetarian food.
- Vegetables, such as beans, peas, cauliflower, mushrooms and spinach.
- Coffee, tea, chocolate and alcohol.
- Reduce whole grains, legumes, milk, cheese, butter and sugar.
- Drinking plenty of water helps in excretion of uric acid.

ARTHRITIS OF THE SHOULDER

Arthritis in the shoulder is uncommon. Pain and loss of movement occur when structures around the joint are affected.

The innervations of the shoulder joint and surrounding structures is mainly through the fifth cervical root (issuing from the vertebrae of the neck), lying in the area of deltoid muscle, extending over the shoulder and upper arm, and hence, pain is often felt over the deltoid region.

Frozen shoulder is the most common ailment in the fifty to seventy years age group, with women affected twice as often as men. The trigger factors are painful external conditions, which lead to immobilisation of the shoulder. These include heart attack, removal of breast, cerebro-vascular accidents or any other major surgery in the chest region.

The ailment starts with pain and soreness in the upper arm, with such increase in severity that it often disturbs sleep.

Osteoarthritis in the shoulder, though rare, is termed as Periarthritis and, at times, crepitating is heard on movements of the shoulder.

Treatment
- Gentle massage to the shoulder area, followed by hot and cold fomentation or affusion.
- Exposing the painful area to infrared rays, followed by cold compresses or direct mud application.
- Cold packs, for forty-five to sixty minutes in the nights, regularly.
- Exercises—movement of the shoulder joints in all directions.

SPINAL PROBLEMS

The spinal column comprises of thirty-three tiny bones, aligned perfectly from the bottom of the skull and running down to the hip region. Spinal cord supports the brain at the top, anchors the rib cage at the centre and joins the pelvis at the bottom. The spine must carry the weight of the human frame, be flexible and allow bending and rotation in all directions, even with heavy load. It should also be hollow to allow delicate nerves and blood vessels to pass through it and emerge from its sides, not be damaged during movement and function adequately for a lifetime.

The individual vertebra is held together by ligaments. The spinal cord travels down a hollow vertebral canal towards the back, sending out nerve roots through openings at the side of each vertebra. The sciatic nerve, which extends from lumbar region supplying to the lower limbs, is often involved in severe backache. Between each vertebra, there is a cushion made of gelatinous centre, called disc, which acts as a shock absorber and can withstand the weight equivalent to the weight of two refrigerators.

Cervical Spondylosis

This is the condition where the bones of the neck (cervical vertebrae) undergo changes of wear and tear. Cervical Spondylosis is more common amongst the aged but that does not mean the younger age group is free from it. In fact, irrespective of age, it is striking all now, which is mainly due to unhealthy lifestyle and the way the spinal cord is used for daily activities. Incorrect posture, whiplash while driving vehicles, constantly bending forward while working, stress and strain—all result in pain and stiffness in the neck region. Apart from pain and stiffness are the radiating pains to shoulder and hands with feeling of pricking of pins and needles and frequent giddiness (due to deficiency in or compression on the basilar artery supplying blood to brain).

Sometimes, Cervical Spondylosis sufferers are advised to wear a collar belt that immobilises the area and provides relief from pain. But absolute immobilisation can lead to permanent stiffness and muscles may become weak.

Treatment
- Avoidance of constant bending forward and pressure over the neck.
- Gentle massage to neck, spine and shoulder, followed by hot and cold affusions or neutral affusion.
- Hot and cold fomentations, in case of acute spasm and pain.
- Arm contrast baths to relieve radiating pain to hands.
- Regular head and neck exercises.
- Maintenance of correct posture during all activities.

Low Backache

Most people suffer from backache at some time or other in their lives. This is the penalty to be paid for assuming wrong posture.

Backache is second only to headache among the leading causes of pain. Most of the backache sufferers otherwise lead a normal life.

Though drugs provide relief from severe pain or relax the muscles, they are not a cure for it. If they are overused, they may become a habit and actually increase the recurrence of pain.

Recurring backache often results in devitalisation, fatigue and depression. This recurrence is quite common amongst the diagnosed low backache sufferers. Psychological stress, a known factor in precipitating backaches, is responsible for stiffness of the back muscles, which then causes painful spasm resulting in backache.

Apart from overuse/misuse of the spine, stress and sedentary habits, other causes of backache include weakened back muscles; protruded abdomen, which pulls back muscles, thereby placing extra stress on the back; overexercising, such as jogging, aerobics, etc.; and Obesity. The aging process also contributes to backache.

In fact, about eighty to eighty-five per cent of backache is due to muscular weakness, stress, etc., and fifteen to twenty per cent as a result of structural defect or diseases, such as Osteoarthritis, prolapsed inter-vertebral disc, Lumbar Spondylosis, Spinal Canal Stenosis, Facet Joint Syndrome and Spondylolisthēsis.

As compared to standing, sitting increases the pressure exerted on the back by forty per cent, while lying down decreases it to twenty-five per cent. Sneezing, laughing and coughing also increase disc pressure and, hence, aggravate the backache.

Treatment

- RICE Principle is to be adopted in case of acute or severe low backache for first twenty-four to forty-eight hours.

  R – Resting the painful area.

  I – Ice-cold packs at repeated intervals.

  C – Cold compresses application frequently.

  E – Elevation of the affected area to help movement of accumulated blood to other areas.

- Gentle, low back massage, followed by hot and cold affusions or fomentation.
- Infrared treatment to the affected area, followed by direct mud application or a cold compress.
- Neutral spinal bath, to relieve pain and numbness in the lower limbs.
- Neutral immersion and half bath with Epsom salt, for ten to twenty minutes.
- Hot hip bath, for ten to twelve minutes, for relieving backache.
- Neutral jet massage, whirlpool baths and underwater massage, to relax the stiff back muscles.
- Steam bath is also useful in providing muscular relaxation due to its thermic effect.
- Regular back-bending exercises, coupled with maintainence of proper back posture, avoidance of lifting heavy weight and sudden jerks.
- Regular practice of breathing exercises help in movement of spinal cord, resulting in relief from referred pains due to the compression on the nerve endings.

Ankylosing Spondylitis

It is an inflammatory disorder of the spinal cord, resulting in fusion of vertebrae due to loose bodies being formed around the structures, causing stiffness and rigidity. Totally-fused spinal cord is quite an advanced stage of the disease and the spinal cord looks like a bamboo stick. Hence, it is also known as Bamboo Spine.

Treatments

Treatments listed for lower and upper backaches hold good for this condition also.

CALCANEAL SPUR

It is a condition occurring due to the deposition of calcium around the calcaneum bone (heel bone), resulting in pain. Pain is particularly felt when the foot is placed on the floor, but disappears after one walks a few steps.

Treatment

- Since excess weight adds to the existing problem, reduction of weight is essential.

- Hot foot immersion with Epsom salt, before going to bed and in the morning, on raising from bed, relieves the pain.

- Wear soft slippers, cushioned at the heel.

Chapter XII

Digestive Diseases

Three entities sustain human life on this planet. They are air, water and food—in that order. The food one eats has to be broken down to yield the much-needed energy and the ingredients of nutrition, like protein, fat, carbohydrates, vitamins and minerals.

Apart from digestion, assimilation and absorption, the digestive system performs another important function, i.e. elimination of wastes accumulated after completion of the above process of digestion.

The digestive process is responsible for converting the food into energy and use/store it for various activities. At the same time, it is quite capable of building up toxins, too. A pioneer English naturopath, Harry Benjamin, rightly said that food, in requisite amounts, yields useful energy for basic life activities, growth and development. On the contrary, body organs and their cells cannot make use of nutrients when their concentration exceeds the set limit. This limit is termed as biological optimum. For example, most people consider it a healthy trait to eat sumptuously at every meal. In fact, it is a wrong practice. Rather, leaving the table with a feeling that the stomach can still take some more is the right kind of practice.

When a person lets whims get the better of him and takes another helping, knowing fully well that he does not need it, he is wantonly allowing accumulation of food. This excess food remains undigested and unutilised, and slowly clogs the intestine, putrefies to produce acids, causing a steady atony of the intestinal musculature and leads to Constipation. And this Constipation is responsible for a great number of physiological derangements, better known to us as diseases.

This vicious chain of acid formation goes on to leave the system in a perpetually unhealthy state of acidity, which is diametrically opposite to the normal, slightly alkaline state of good health. Such Constipation eventually renders the nutritive system a troublesome brewpot of acid residues, which is detrimental to good health. But note, once it is allowed to set in, Constipation stays on to become chronic, resulting in accumulation of waste food leading to putrefaction, and the inevitable formation of toxins in the bloodstream. Meanwhile, the putrefying wastes in the intestines serve as a sub-strata for pathogens (disease-causing micro-organisms) and making it a breeding ground for serious forms of fever and acute disorders.

The overlying acidity and the underlying chronic Constipation, together form a Pandora's Box. The resulting disease depends on the resistance an individual has built up.

So, essentially, it is the food we eat and how much we eat that forms the root cause of various ailments, generally labelled as digestive disorders. Let us, therefore, now look at each of them in detail.

HYPERACIDITY

Excessive consumption of sugar and starch leads to production of fermented acids in the digestive system. The excess acid flushes into the bloodstream, making it hypo-alkaline. Another cause of Hyperacidity is missing a meal in between or not taking it at fixed intervals, resulting in hypersecretion of acid in the stomach, which burns its soft, delicate, mucosal lining. At times, the acid regurgitates into the oesophagus, and causes a burning sensation in the throat region (heartburn). Intake of spicy food, stimulants such as coffee, tea, alcohol, smoking, tobacco chewing and stress and strains, all directly result in hypersecretion of hydrochloric acid in the stomach.

Treatment

- Routine treatments like mudpacks or cold compresses on the abdomen, twice a day, or cold hip baths, daily.

- Hot and cold fomentations to abdomen, once in a while.

- Cold abdominal pack every night.

- Kidney pack, once in a while.

- Well-planned meals of fixed quantity at fixed timings.

- Adequate intake of water.

- Cold trunk pack, once in a while.

- Taking enema for three days at the beginning of the treatment, to cleanse the intestine of morbid matter.

ULCERS

Ulcers are caused by the erosion of the inner, mucosal lining of the stomach due to excessive secretion of acid. As popularly known to mankind, "Hurry, Worry and Curry" combination heralds the onset of this affliction.

Apart from Hyperacidity, many other physical causes, such as wrong eating habits, irregular meal spacing, spicy food, stimulants, such as tea, coffee, alcohol, tobacco chewing, smoking, stress—physical, emotional and/or psychological—result in Ulcers.

If the erosion of mucus membrane takes place around the stomach, it is termed as Gastric Ulcer, and if in duodenum, it is called Duodenal Ulcer.

Ulcers result in a burning sensation and a gnawing type of pain on empty stomach. It is relieved immediately after ingestion of food or about two hours after its intake. This typical pain-food-relief is the most common symptom of Ulcer.

Treatment

- To begin with, cold milk at regular intervals.

- Later on, fixed meal at regular intervals, which should be free from spices, stimulants, citrus fruits and their juices, non-vegetarian food, raw salads, unripe fruits, etc.

- Cold water enema, taken for a few days, helps to get rid of all accumulated waste.

- Cold abdominal pack everyday.

- Gastro-hepatic pack provides relief from pain.

- Mudpacks to abdomen reduce fermentation and eliminate gas.

- Daily cold hip baths are also recommended.

- Ice applications to abdomen, and kidney pack in case of burning sensation.

- Physical and mental rest.

FLATULENT DYSPEPSIA

Distension or bloating of the abdomen after consumption of food, eructation of gastric fluid and burning sensation in the region of the stomach and chest are all due to Flatulant Dyspepsia. It is not merely a problem in the physiology of digestion, but also that affecting the process of food absorption.

The stomach is, in fact, a temporary storehouse of food, with food in a half digested state, consisting of proteins in the process of digestion, untouched fats and almost fully-digested carbohydrates. The hydrochloric acid destroys harmful, infectious organisms and acts as a protective barrier in the stomach.

The stomach has the capacity to adapt to maximum variations in the food habits of individuals—ranging from all types of sweet, hot, spicy, rich, non-vegetarian, vegetarian foods to beverages like coffee, tea and alcoholic drinks. But if people are unable to digest certain foodstuffs, such as milk, fish, meat and egg, it leads to indigestion.

Indigestion leads to gas formation, accompanied by a feeling of bloating or distention, pain or passing flatus or even both.

Belching, another symptom of gas formation, is mainly due to swallowing too much of air while drinking or eating, inappropriate relaxation of the lower oesophageal opening, resulting in gastro-oesophaeal reflux.

Treatment

- Relax and eat slowly; both, the physical state of food and the mental state of a person are equally important.
- Drink warm water to eliminate gases.
- Avoid fatty foods, tea, coffee, citrus fruits and their juices, alcohol, smoking and high protein diet.
- Hot and cold fomentation helps in relieving gas and pain in the abdomen.
- Gastro-hepatic pack provides relief from pains.
- Cold abdominal pack, forty-five to sixty minutes daily.
- Enema, for first couple of days, to cleanse the system.
- Mudpacks to improve blood circulation to the abdominal region.
- Lying down on the abdomen and practice of pavanmuktasana.
- Replacement of the intestinal flora by reducing fat and protein and increasing the intake of non-fat curd and butter-milk.

GASTRITIS

Gastritis causes a range of disorders that affect the very process of good ingestion. Nausea, bloating of stomach, eructation, gas, pain, burning sensation and generalised malaise after the intake of food. It occurs on account of inflammation of the stomach's delicate, inner mucosal lining. Vomiting of partly-digested food and passing of blood-tinged or blood in stools sometimes, are some of the symptoms of Gastritis.

The causes can range from excessive drug intake to physical and mental stress.

Treatment

- Enema, for two to three days, to cleanse the system, and later on, as and when required.
- Mudpack to improve circulation to abdominal organs, once in every two to three hours.
- Cold hip bath daily.
- Gastro-hepatic pack to reduce pain.

- Cold abdominal pack everyday.

- Hot and cold fomentation to abdomen.

- Hot and cold hip bath on alternate days.

- Avoidance of food, except ice-cold milk at regular intervals, till symptoms persist. Sucking on ice cubes may help.

- Once the acute symptoms disappear, steps to reduce mucosal irritation should be taken. Dietary regulations, such as small meals at fixed timings should be followed. Also, avoiding of irritants (drugs, coffee, alcohol, smoking, etc.) is important.

DISORDERS OF THE SMALL INTESTINE

As we move down from the stomach, we reach the small intestine, which is divided into three portions: Duodenum, Jejunum and Ileum.

Partially-digested proteins, almost-digested carbohydrates and untouched fats pass on to the intestine from the stomach. Here, they are digested completely with the help of intestinal juice, which is a combination of intestinal secretion, bile acids and pancreatic juice. After the digestion, absorption takes place in the ileum (the last part), through specialised structures called villi. If the absorptive pathway is not all that smooth, then several disorders affect the intestines, such as Duodenitis, Enteric Fever, Typhoid, Malabsorption Syndrome (Tropical Sprue), etc.

Duodenitis

As in Gastritis, in Duodenitis also the delicate, mucosal lining of the intestine is inflamed. The resultant problems are same as in Gastritis, except for the pain, which is felt a little to the right and above the navel rather than the stomach itself. If it is ignored, it may lead to Duodenal Ulceration, or if it spreads to the other parts of the intestines, it may cause Enteritis.

Treatment

- Cold compress and Mudpacks are routinely applied to improve blood circulation to abdominal region and to check intestinal fermentation.

- Cold hip bath, for twenty minutes everyday, ensures better muscular functioning in the digestive region.

- Periodic, short fasts, with adequate water intake and required precaution will improve digestive and absorptive capacity of the intestinal region.

- Cold water enema, for two to three days, to cleanse the system.

- Hot and cold compress, hot and cold alternate hip bath and gastro-hepatic packs provide relief from pains.

- Abdominal pack before going to bed acts as a tonic.

- Milk diet, to start with, and later on, non-spicy, non-irritant, bland diet at regular intervals.

DISORDER OF THE LARGE INTESTINE

The large intestine (colon) is responsible for absorbing water from the end products of digestion and eliminating the wastes. A diet with adequate quantity of water is essential to perform this important function of the large intestine. A diet which is low in fibre content does immense harm. At times, instead of drying up the waste food, known as faeces, the colon induces frequent passage of stool, with large amounts of water, resulting in Diarrhoea. Chronic Constipation is actually said to be the root cause of Diarrhoea. The large intestine, being blocked with accumulated faeces, triggers the body's healing mechanism to induce an acute disorder so that the system is cleansed. However, if properly attended to, the symptoms could be taken care of in a day or two, without any complications.

Colitis

Colitis is inflammation of the colon and is of two types—mucus and ulcerative. It can occur both in adults and children. Though the exact cause of this problem is not known, in a typical case of Ulcerative Colitis, lining of "crypts" (tubular depression in the colon) is involved. The crypts break down and purulent effusion fills them. The mucus membrane is inflamed and swollen, and the damage may slowly spread to the deeper layers of the intestine. This effectively reduces the diameter of the large intestine, resulting in abnormal constriction. This results in difficulty in evacuation of wastes, causing pain and passing, six to twelve times, loose stools, with blood and mucus. It causes weight loss, and in a few cases, it may be severe.

Treatment

Soothing diet for three to six months at least, consisting of soft, cooked vegetables, rice or dal and well-ripened fruits like banana and papaya. Tender coconut water is soothing to the soft mucosa of the colon. Cooked (boiled or baked) apples aid in healing.

- Repeated application of mudpacks on the abdomen, several times a day.
- Tonic exercise with cold water.
- Enema with butter-milk, instead of water, helps reinstate healthy flora of the colon.

Diverticulitis

The intestine possesses several pouches or sac-like structures along its course, called diverticulae. When undigested waste matter stagnates in one or several such diverticula, the mucosal lining of the colon suffers inflammation and presents symptoms of acute and chronic Diverticulitis.

The usual symptoms of Diverticulitis are cramping pain in the left, lower abdomen and Constipation, alternating with Diarrhoea. There may be irritation of the peritoneum, Fever, chills, Peritonitis or abscess.

Treatment

- Mudpacks to abdomen or cold compresses.
- Cold hip bath daily.
- Alternate hip bath, two to three times a week.
- Abdominal pack every night.
- Gastro-hepatic pack, two or three times a week.
- Regular enema treatment, initially, and then tapering off as diet and exercise show their effects.
- Fasting, initially for two to three days, followed by a fruit and raw vegetable diet for a few days. A high fibre diet to be introduced gradually.

- Intake of fluid in plenty.
- Regular physical exercises.
- Regular, early morning toilet training.
- Adjustment to emotional disturbances.

DIARRHOEA

Diarrhoea is a condition where there is an increase in the frequency, fluidity (water content) and volume of stool. When the colon is unable to carry out its set job of absorbing water from undigested wastes, there occurs the common complaint of excessive presence of water in stools and frequent passage of loose stools. The cause is either an impairment in the absorptive capacity of the large intestine or a combined malfunctioning of the absorptive action of the small intestine and other digestive organs.

From principles of naturopathy, Diarrhoea is a naturally induced phenomenon that calls for a rapid expulsion of waste.

Treatment
- Ice-cold water enemas, for first couple of days.
- Mudpacks/towelpacks, at an interval of every two hours.
- Complete fasting on butter-milk and tender coconut water, and drinking plenty of water, initially for two to three days. Drinking copious water is necessary to maintain the water content of the body.
- After two to three days of fast, a diet comprising of sabudana kheer, curd rice, well-ripened banana and butter-milk should be taken till symptoms last.

Chronic Amoebiasis

It is a widely prevalent disease, brought about by unhygienic habits and insanitary conditions.

Amoebiasis is due to a single-cell organism called Entamoeba hystolitica, which gains entry into the body either through contaminated drinking water or food. After getting entry, it lodges itself in the large intestine, forming cysts.

Symptoms like Dyspepsia, flatulence, nausea, heartburn and occasional loose motions, often accompanied by a feeling of ill-health, are quite common. In severe cases, there will be increased frequency of stools with blood and mucus, fever, vomiting, etc.

If untreated, it may lead to amoebic liver and lung abscess.

Treatment

- Fasting, initially for two to three days.
- Warm neem water enema, for the first three days.
- Cold hip bath daily.
- Mudpacks, at regular intervals, for twenty minutes, depending on severity.
- Kidney pack, once or twice a week.
- Abdominal pack daily.
- Gastro-hepatic pack to relieve distention and pain.
- Hot and cold fomentation to abdomen, hot and cold hip bath, once a while.

Constipation

Constipation is an altered function of the bowels, where they are emptied at a longer interval than normally required, with or without any difficulty.

It is a common affliction of modern civilisation, caused due to unhealthy lifestyle. The incidence of Constipation in the general population is variable. Most people pass one or two motions per day and it is considered to be normal. But more than three bowel movements a day may be termed abnormal. Majority of the people are quite obsessed with the number and frequency of the bowel action. They often exhibit a sense of concern when either the amount of stool passed is too little or if there is a feeling of inadequate evacuation.

Constipation may be due to a number of factors, such as inadequate intake of fluids, absence of roughage in the diet, lack of regular exercise, faulty food intake, not attending to nature's call in time, etc.

Treatment
(Same as that for Diverticulitis.)

Chapter XIII

Respiratory Diseases

Almost everyone, at one time or the other, suffers from cold, running nose, blocked nostrils, heaviness in the head and other common respiratory tract problems. By taking care of these acute respiratory problems/infections early, one can prevent more serious respiratory tract illnesses, such as Bronchitis, Bronchial Asthma, Emphysema, etc.

COMMON COLD

It is an exceedingly common respiratory infection. It is due to a virus which multiplies fast in a person whose vitality is low. The cold is, in fact, nature's simplest mechanism of eliminating wastes accumulated in the system—popularly known as "healing crisis".

ALLERGIC RHINITIS (HAY FEVER)

Watery, nasal discharge, sneezing, itching of eyes and nose, and increased eosinophil count in blood are common features of Allergic Rhinitis. Like the common cold, it is self-limiting (does not run a long course in one episode) in nature.

Treatment

The body's immunity (resistance) should be improved by cleaning the internal system with a short fast of three days or till the symptoms last, along with regular warm water enemas early in the morning.

- Gargling frequently with warm, salt or honey water soothes the throat.

- Drinking plenty of warm water with honey and ginger or tulsi water with honey causes counter-irritation, providing relief from sore throat.

- Hot foot and arm bath, which relieves congestion in the head region, provides relief from heaviness in the head and other symptoms of cold.

- Generally, secretions of the nasal passages are slightly acidic, but during cold they become alkaline. Their acidity can be maintained by inhaling steam. Eucalyptus oil or camphor can be added to the water used for this purpose.

- Throat pack, at night, till symptoms of sore throat persist, is also an effective measure.

- Steam/sauna bath, twice a week, facilitates elimination.

- Jalaneti and sutraneti help to clear the nasal secretions and opening the nasal passages.

- To prevent frequent attacks of Cold/Rhinitis, one should regularly take adequate quantities of Vitamin C, which improves one's resistance. Citrus fruit juices, such as lemon, orange, sweet lime and Indian gooseberries are excellent sources of Vitamin C. Fruits, such as guava, are also fair sources of Vitamin C.

RECURRENT LARYNGITIS, TONSILLITIS

Laryngitis and Tonsillitis are inflammation of the larynx (wind pipe) and tonsils, respectively. In both the cases, there will be pain, sore throat, low degree fever and malaise, all of which generally persist for a few days. Like Cold and Rhinitis, both the conditions are self-limiting in nature.

Treatment

- Hot foot and arm baths, three days continuously at the beginning, and twice a week later.

- Enema, daily, for three days, and mud pack to abdomen, daily.

- Throat packs for forty-five to sixty minutes, till the symptoms last.

- Hot and cold fomentation to the throat and steam inhalation daily (thrice), to provide symptomatic relief.

- Fasting with fruit juice, lemon juice or vegetable soups until symptoms subside.

- Warm, saline water or honey water gargling provides soothing effect and also helps in clearing mucus from throat region.

- Taking plenty of warm, honey water with ginger juice causes counter-irritation, providing relief and foments the region, relieving pain.

SINUSITIS

Sinuses are paired, hollow spaces connected with the nasal passages arranged in the skull region. There are frontal, maxillary, ethmoid and sphenoid sinuses. Since they are connected to the nasal passages, any infection to the nose and throat region can spread to them. Thus, secretions accumulate in the sinuses, resulting in heaviness in the head, blocked nostrils, nasal discharge, and pain and tenderness in the area of involved sinus.

Treatment

- Fasting on fruit juices or lemon juice till symptoms last forms an important part of the treatment.

- Enema, successively for three days, and later on, as required. Mudpack on abdomen, twice daily.

- Cold friction bath and immersion bath activates the skin, thus relieving the sinuses.

- Massage over the sinus region helps in draining out the accumulated mucus.

- Hot foot and arm bath diverts blood supply to the upper and lower limbs. This relieves pressure on the inflamed sinuses, providing relief from heaviness and pain.

- Steam inhalation, by boiling water with Eucalyptus leaves or camphor, helps in draining out nasal secretions and opening up blocked nostrils.

- Jalaneti and sutraneti also help in clearing nasal secretions, thus facilitating easier breathing.
- Steam/sauna bath help in clearing the congestion of sinuses.
- Smelling freshly chopped onions, sometimes, opens up the clogged nasal passages.
- Fomentation over the sinuses area also gives immense relief.

BRONCHITIS

Acute Bronchitis

Inflammation of the bronchioles (small air passages or tubes in the lung) due to untreated upper respiratory infection can result in acute Bronchitis. This causes cough with sputum, sore throat, low degree fever and heaviness in the chest.

Chronic Bronchitis

It is often termed as Chronic Obstructive Pulmonary Disease (COPD). It is a progressive disease, affecting the mucus membrane of the bronchi. For many, Bronchitis is the result of long exposure to irritants like cotton dust, silica, smoking, recurrent viral or bacterial infection (as in recurrent acute Bronchitis) and changes in temperature.

Initially, the patient will have more problem during winter, with cough, sputum, breathlessness and a feeling of tightness in the chest. This gradually increases in severity and duration, resulting in persistent cough with large quantity of sputum. The sputum will be more in the morning. Occasionally, wheezing occurs along with the feeling of tightness. The sputum is a thick, sticky (mucoid), thread-like substance and may be yellow if infection is superadded.

Asthma

There are two types of asthma patients—those who would like to know everything about asthma and those who are irresponsibly ignorant about it. A patient who is not properly informed about the disease and its consequences has a poor prognosis.

Asthma occurs in the form of attacks of coughing, wheezing and breathlessness and is completely reversible. The duration of attack varies. It may occur during certain seasons or with seasonal changes or might even persist throughout the year.

The specific cause of asthma is not known. It is observed that asthma begins in the childhood itself in majority of cases and, in most bronchial asthma sufferers, there will be a family history of allergy. The allergy may manifest as Rhinitis, Eczema or Urticarial Rash or Asthma. If both parents suffer from some form of allergy, the chances of their child developing Asthma at a young age is greater.

In some cases, Asthma starts at a late age and is often not associated with a specific allergic or triggering factor.

Long-standing cases of Bronchial Asthma may result in many complications, especially if inadequately treated.

Emphysema, a permanent destruction of alveolar air spaces resulting in reduced elastic recoil of lungs, is the most common complication. Corpulmonale, where the heart is also involved, is another complication.

Children face the problem of stunted growth and are more prone to rib fractures. Most patients with Bronchial Asthma adjust very well and continue to lead a normal life, if early indications of the attack are properly treated. Hence, thorough education of the patient about the disease goes a long way in the treatment of asthma.

Treatment of Bronchial Asthma in an Impending Attack

- Not to panic, for anxiety will only accentuate the attack.
- Rest and relaxation. Sit down on a chair for 10 minutes, as resting helps lungs to relax. Breathe slowly, taking small puffs of air through pursed lips.
- One should take rest in a warm, well-ventilated room.
- Bedclothes should be warm.
- Patient should be supported by pillows in a semi-recumbent or upright position.

- Fasting with vegetable soup and hot, honey water is helpful.

- Take enema. Emptying bowel will relieve pressure on the lungs.

- Plenty of warm liquids relax the air passages by fomenting the wind pipe (which is in front of the food pipe). Liquids also thin the mucus and replace the water lost during forced breathing.

- Gentle, spinal massage, followed by hot fomentation to back and neutral chest pack, helps in relaxing the bronchial muscles. Hot fomentation softens the mucus and chest pack relieves congestion in the lungs.

- Try exhaling forcefully through a drinking straw inserted into a large bottle of water. The resistance of the water will force the expansion of bronchial tubes by creating positive pressure in the lungs.

- Facial steam will clear upper respiratory secretions.

- Hot foot and arm bath relieves congestion by diverting blood flow to limbs.

Long Term Treatment of Acute Bronchitis / Chronic Bronchitis / Bronchial Asthma
Besides the above-mentioned measures, following are also to be adopted.

- Treat fever by means of freqeunt sponge baths, chest packs every night and friction baths.

- Patient should refrain from smoking.

- Practice of jalaneti and sutraneti, as and when required, keeps upper respiratory passages clear.

- Neutral half baths with Epsom salt, which divert blood to the periphery and relieve lung congestion, could be employed frequently with advantage.

- Asthma bath, once a week or 15 days, is useful in relieving congestion and increasing oxygen consumption.

- Neutral underwater massage, neutral jet massage and whirlpool bath provide relaxaion by acting on the muscles in the spinal region.
- A mucusless diet to be adopted.
- Pranayama and asanas help build resistance of the lung and upper respiratory tract, besides clearing them.

Chapter XIV

Cardiovascular System Diseases

HYPERTENSION

Hypertension (high blood pressure) is a resultant disease of the modern society. The present day socio-economic culture, very often, stretches personal and social life beyond one's tolerance limit. This creates ground for many diseases, chief among which is Hypertension.

At present, Hypertension is prevailing in almost one-seventh of the population of the world's industrially developed countries. As the disease strikes lethal blows without giving any warming, it is aptly termed as a "silent killer".

Ironically, of all the known ailments that lead to premature deaths, Hypertension is the easiest to control.

The pressure required to pump blood evenly to all parts of the body is called blood pressure. It normally ranges between 110/60 mm Hg to 140/85 mm Hg. If pressure consistently rises beyond 140/85 mm Hg on three different times, then one is considered to be hypertensive.

The cause of essential Hypertension (where blood pressure is raised without any primary cause, in the heart, kidneys and adrenal glands) is still unknown. Depending on its level of rise, blood pressure is categorised as mild, moderate or severe Hypertension.

Sudden rise in blood pressure and severe, uncontrolled Hypertension may lead to complications, such as paralytic stroke, heart attack, congestive heart failure, kidney failure and even blindness, due to detachment of retina.

Maintaining blood pressure at a safe level should be the aim of every hypertensive individual. This requires a little sacrifice and the determination to abide by restrictions.

Treatment

Blood pressure is normally within safe limits by the following factors:

1. Pumping action of the heart.
2. Elasticity of the blood vessels.
3. Quality of blood flowing in the bloodstream.
4. Viscosity (thickness) of blood.
5. Peripheral arterial resistance.

Most of the above factors can be taken care of by following a drugless method.

The quality of blood can be improved by following a strict regimen of diet, which comprises:

i) Caloric restriction, if overweight.

ii) 10-15% fat, 60-70% carbohydrate and 15-20% protein.

iii) Low in cholesterol.

iv) Low in salt, which helps eliminate excess water.

v) Increased dietary fibre.

Treatment, such as neutral half bath, neutral half bath with friction and Epsom salt, and steam baths (in case of mild Hypertension), result in peripheral vasodilation, which relaxes the heart muscle and improves peripheral arterial resistance. By means of hot and cold water treatments, blood circulation to the periphery, as well as to the internal organs, could be improved. Through such treatments, popularly known as "vascular training", the elasticity (constriction and relaxation) of the blood vessels can be improved.

- Cold spinal bath, ice massage to the head and spine, troma and cold pack to head, cold friction, sponge bath, mudbath and cold chest packs, all help in bringing down the blood pressure immediately.

- Mudpacks applied to abdomen, regularly, improve circulation of blood to the abdominal region.

- Full body massages, done in reverse direction, once or twice a week, not only relax the skeletal muscles, but also improve peripheral circulation and lymphatic drainage.

Yoga therapy, which comprises of yogic kriyas, pranayama, asanas and yoganidra, helps in cleansing the internal system, improving immunity, functioning capacity of the internal organs, providing flexibility, agility, endurance and also a deep sense of relaxation. The heart muscle, when relaxed, reduces pulse rate, heartbeat and blood pressure.

Like any other chronic disease, Hypertension is to be treated throughout. By following above norms, blood pressure can be maintained at a safe level always.

VARICOSE VEINS

Varicose Veins are irregularly dilated, lengthened and thickened veins. They may appear on any part of the body—the oesophageal, haemorrhoidal and spermatic veins—but most commonly in the legs. Approximately twenty per cent of the population of developed countries have Varicose Veins in their legs. Women are more prone to it than men (ratio 5:1) and the left leg is more commonly affected than right by this disease. Sixty-six per cent of sufferers usually have a strong family history of Varicose Veins.

Veins are the vessels or tubes that carry the blood back to the heart. They have valves, which ensure the flow of blood only in one direction. When veins dilate, their valves become incompetent, resulting in pooling and stagnation of blood in the superficial veins. Consequently, the water in the stagnated and pooled blood rushes to tissue spaces in the leg, leading to oedema (swelling), and later on to other complications, such as pigmentation of skin (discolouration), fat necrosis (destruction of fatty tissue), Eczema, and finally, Ischaemia (lack of blood supply) and ulceration.

Varicose Veins is usually seen amongst people who work standing or sitting for long periods of time. Traffic policemen, teachers and people practicing other such vocation, and sedentary workers are more prone to the problem. Gravitational pull, obesity and hormonal influences aggravate the problem.

Varicose Veins results in pain, fatigue and heaviness in the legs, ankle swelling, cramps in the legs—especially at night, pigmentation of skin, Stasis Dermatitis, Cellulitis of lower limb, etc.

Treatment

- Reduction of weight, if overweight.
- Avoid standing or sitting for long hours.
- Neutral immersion bath with Epsom salt.
- Contrast foot bath (alternate hot and cold), periodically, to relieve cramps, aches and pains.
- Cold packs to the legs, applied every night, are also beneficial.
- Direct mud application to the legs, once in a while (if there is no ulceration).
- Elevation of affected leg with the help of pillows. By reducing gravitational pull, venous drainage is improved.
- Drink plenty of tender coconut water, barley water, dhania water or cucumber juice—all without salt—to remove excess water from the system.
- Wear elastic stockings if prolonged standing or sitting cannot be avoided. They help to compress the varicosed veins.
- Regular exercises, such as contracting leg muscles, help the movement of stagnant blood in the veins.
- Walking or treading in cold water relieves painful swelling of veins. The massaging effect due to movement in water helps in stimulating nerve endings around the blood vessels.

Chapter XV

Menstrual Disorders

Menstruation, which marks the end of ovulation cycle in non-pregnant female primates, begins around puberty and stops at around the age of forty-five years. Menstrual disorders that commonly occur are Dysfunctional Uterine Bleeding (DUB), premenstrual syndrome, post-menopausal bleeding, debilitating, and occasionally, even critical.

PATTERNS OF ABNORMAL UTERINE BLEEDING

Menorrhagia: Excessive bleeding, but the menstrual cycle may be of normal length.

Polymenorrhoea: Episodes of bleeding occurring in less than twenty-one days.

Oligomenorrhoea: Scanty menstruation.

Metrorrhagia: Irregular uterine bleeding at any time between menstrual periods.

PREMENSTRUAL SYNDROME (PMS)

Approximately forty per cent of menstruating women suffer from premenstrual syndrome, which tends to occur three to seven days prior to the menstrual period. The symptoms include headaches, nausea, irritability, fatigue, bloating in abdomen, oedema in feet and hands, craving for sweets, depression and tenderness in breast. These symptoms generally disappear with the onset of menstruation.

Treatment
- Sympathetic understanding, reassurance with the help of behaviour therapist or psychologist.

101

- A well-balanced diet with restriction on salt, as water retention is quite common before the onset of menstruation.

- Use of tender coconut water, barley water, dhania water or butter-milk has a diuretic effect.

- Adequate rest and relaxation is essential. Practising yoganidra or shavasana, for ten minutes regularly, is beneficial.

- Headaches can be relieved by dry head massage followed by hot foot immersion, for twenty minutes.

- Facial steam, for five to ten minutes regularly, helps in providing relief from headaches.

- Warm water bath provides relaxation and relieves fatigue and irritation.

- Drinking a glass of warm milk with honey helps in getting good sleep.

Treatment for Excessive Menstruation (Menorrhagia, Polymenorrhea)

- Wet girdle pack at night, daily, for one hour.

- Ice-cold mudpacks applied on the lower abdomen at repeated intervals help check bleeding.

- Absolute bed-rest, with leg elevated in an ideal posture during Menorrhagia.

- Cold foot and arm baths, taken frequently, constrict the blood vessels supplying pelvic organs, thereby reducing the bleeding.

- Preventive measures like a well-balanced diet, adequate rest, relaxation and regular physical exercises, such as walking, yoga, pranayama, should be a part of the treatment.

- All other treatments which improve general health (mentioned in the previous chapters) hold good here also.

- If bleeding continues even after symptomatic treatments, medical intervention is very essential. A gynaecologist should be consulted immediately.

DYSMENORRHOEA

Pain that occurs during menstruation is common in about sixty per cent of menstruating women. Sometimes, it is severe enough to interfere with normal daily activity.

Primary Dysmenorrhoea

It occurs only in the absence of pelvic disease. It usually starts two to three years after the onset of menstruation and worsens between the age of seventeen to twenty-four years, and then subsides on its own.

Secondary Dysmenorrhoea

Secondary Dysmenorrhoea is generally due to a definite cause, such as pelvic inflammation, fibroid in the uterus, Endometriosis, tumours of the ovary, or even presence of an intrauterine device. In all such cases of Dysmenorrhoea, where the definite cause is known, medical intervention to correct the underlying defect will provide relief from pain.

Treatment

- Cold hip bath, daily, for ten to fifteen minutes, cures all menstrual disorders.
- Proper, regulated, well-balanced diet.
- Regular physical excercises, except during the periods.
- Absolute bed-rest with slight elevation of both legs while lying down and a warm water bath during painful episodes of menstruation.
- Hot fomentation to lower abdomen if bleeding is not excessive, to relieve crampy abdominal pain.
- Hot and cold hip baths or compresses to help dilate the cervix to facilitate smooth flow of menstrual blood and relieve pain, only if bleeding is not excessive.
- Constipation, if present, should be relieved by means of enema.

LEUCORRHOEA

Leucorrhoea is not a disease, but the manifestation of ovulation or a local or systemic disease leading to a discharge of whitish substance, which can occur at any age and affects almost all women some time or the other.

The discharge often gives a strong, offensive odour and can be a source of embarrassment to the woman suffering from it.

The discharge is usually without discomfort, but may result in an itching sensation in and around the genitalia.

Treatment
- Maintenance of good hygiene of the external genitalia, with regular washing with warm water or neem water, is very essential.
- Use of sanitary napkins and tampons reduce soiling of the genitalia, odour and itching.
- Warm water hip baths, for fifteen to twenty minutes, with either neem water or Epsom salt, also provide relief from itching.
- Vaginal douche with neem water prevents infection of the internal organs, reversing Leucorrhoea.
- All other measures mentioned in the previous chapters, to improve general health can also be implemented in the treatment of Leucorrhoea.
- Wet girdle pack at night, for an hour, tones up the uterus.

Chapter XVI

Uro-Genital Disorders

THE URINARY TRACT

The kidneys, ureters, urinary bladder and the urethra constitute this tract. Each of the two kidneys in the body possess over twenty million functional units called nephrons, which filter the blood, removing from it about twenty-two litres of fluid urine for final excretion. The ureters connect the kidneys to the urinary bladder, which stores urine until excretion via the urethra.

Urinary Symptoms

Infection, inflammation and obstruction produce symptoms associated with urination.

- Frequency, urgency and urination at night are common symptoms in urinary tract infection.

- Dysuria (painful urination) and burning pain in the urethra on urination are associated with bladder and prostate gland problems.

- Enuresis (bed-wetting) may be due to urinary tract infection or psychological reasons.

- Urinary incontinence. It may be due to structural defect in the kidneys, urinary tract or physical stress, the urgency associated with infection or dribbling of urine associated with over-distended bladder.

URINARY TRACT INFECTION (UTI)

UTI may be classified as upper (when the kidneys are involved) or lower (when the bladder or urethra are involved). Both require immediate medical intervention.

UTIs tend to recur frequently due to several factors, such as poor hygiene of the genital tract, pregnancy, stone formation in the tract, diabetes and obstruction in the tract, controlling the urge of urination (leading to stagnation of urine) etc.

Infections where kidneys are involved, such as Pyelonephritis and Glomerulonephritis, lead to serious consequences like acute or chronic kidney failure where medical intervention becomes essential.

Treatment

All other infections of the ureters, urethra and bladder can be treated, rather, prevented by certain measures mentioned below:

- Adequate fluid intake and strict checking of input and output of fluids. Drinking eight to ten glasses of water per day would be adequate.

- Proper genital hygiene while using public toilets and latrines to be followed.

- Special care is to be taken during pregnancy.

- Fasting for two to three days, with adequate fluid intake, will reverse the infection.

- Mudpacks over the lower abdomen, at regular intervals, will help to reduce inflammation and irritation.

- Treatment of fever by cold friction baths, sponge baths or regular application of chest packs and cold compresses on the forehead.

- Warm water hip bath, for fifteen to twenty minutes, provides relief from pain and burning sensation.

- Wet girdle pack, twice or thrice a day, during an acute phase of infection, and later, once before going to bed, should be adopted.

- Use kidney packs to improve urinary excretion.

- Taking plenty of tender coconut water, barley water, dhania water or butter-milk is beneficial as they act as diuretics.

PROSTATE GLAND ENLARGEMENT

The prostate gland surrounds the male urinary bladder and the first part of urethra. Enlargement of prostate is quite common among men aged above sixty years. But it is mandatory always to find out the type of enlargement. Most of the prostate enlargements are usually benign (harmless). But biopsy of the enlarged mass will confirm the type of enlargement, i.e. whether it is benign or malignant (cancerous).

Typical features of prostate enlargement are, increased frequency of urination, especially at night, poor stream, hesitancy and urgency.

Treatment

If symptoms are not very severe, then the following simple measures could be employed for relief.

- Adequate intake of water, i.e. roughly eight to ten glasses a day.
- A well-balanced diet comprising of fruits and vegetable salads.
- Constipation should be treated promptly, otherwise the load in the rectum aggravates the problem.
- Hot Epsom salt baths are beneficial.
- Hot and cold hip baths, fifteen to twenty minutes, are also beneficial.
- Hot fomentation to bladder area often helps in free flow of urine.
- Kidney pack, to increase fluid output, should be employed two to three times a week.
- Wet girdle pack application, twice or thrice a day, helps to reduce the swelling of the prostate gland.
- Prostate massage also helps to reduce swelling.
- Drinking barley water, dhania water, tender coconut water or butter-milk helps in free flow of urine.
- One should not drink fluids after eight at night.

Chapter XVII

The Nervous System Disorders

INSOMNIA

The most common disorder of sleep is Insomnia or sleeplessness.

Twice as many women as men complain of Insomnia, and it is more prevalent amongst the elderly. There are three kinds of Insomnia:

- Difficulty in falling asleep

- Waking up in the middle of the night

- Early morning awakening

Insomnia is mainly due to psychiatric or medical problems, such as depression, alcoholism, sleep apnea, nocturnal enuresis (bed-wetting), restless leg syndrome (muscular cramps of calf muscles). Other factors, such as stress and bereavement also lead to temporary Insomnia (about three to four weeks). Fasting and indigestion, too, cause disturbances in sleep.

A small percentage of the disorders of sleeplessness starts during childhood.

Generally, sleep disturbances result in fatigue, irritability and unpredictable work efficiency.

On an average, an adult requires about six to eight hours of sleep a day for proper functioning of the body.

Measures to be Taken for Good Sleep
- To go to bed only when feeling sleepy.

- Not to stay in bed for longer than ten minutes if unable to sleep.

- Not to sleep during the day.

- Try to sleep and get up at the same hour everyday.

- Eat a light, early dinner. At least a three-hour gap should be there between supper and going to bed.

- Take hot and cold foot bath, which relieves cramps occurring in the legs due to Varicose Veins or any other condition.

- Do deep breathing exercises for ten minutes.

- Perform yoganidra or progressive muscular relaxation before going to bed.

- Drink a glass of warm milk or water with honey, or a glass of warm water before going to bed.

- Avoid stimulating drinks, such as coffee, tea, cola or cocoa with evening meals or later.

- Take hot foot immersion bath, for twenty to thirty minutes, or prolonged cold foot bath, for forty-five to sixty minutes.

- Cold spinal bath is a tonic that induces sleep.

- Massage, taken twice or thrice a week, is helpful in inducing sleep.

HEADACHE

Headaches affect people of all ages, occupation, caste, creed and race. It has become a part and parcel of one's daily life. Headaches can occur due to emotional disorders, head injuries, Migraine, Fever, intracranial vascular disorders, dental diseases, diseases of the eyes, ears, nose or even sinuses. However, a majority of the headaches are due to modernisation and our changed lifestyle and habits, such as improper diet, tension, stress, sedentary habits, smoking, alcohol, consumption of stimulants, such as coffee and tea. Headaches, in fact, are a distress signal sent up by the body, indicating that all is not well with the system. However, many headache sufferers do not think so and try to suppress it with analgesics, while continuing with unhealthy lifestyle, resulting in the manifestation of another bout of headache soon.

Most people experience headache as a sort of "pain in the head", which is actually due to congestion in the blood vessels that press the nerve endings present in the skull region.

Depending on the cause, headaches are classified as tension headaches, toxaemic headaches, congestive headaches, sinus headaches, postural headaches, cluster headaches and one-sided headache (otherwise known as migraine).

Treatment

- Since Constipation is the root cause of most of the simple forms of headaches, treat Constipation.

- Take warm water enema.

- Do kunjal kriya (induce vomiting) to cleanse the upper gastric region so that pressure is relieved.

- A gentle head, neck and trapezius region massage, followed by cold troma and pack, gives relief.

- Hot foot bath, diverting blood to lower limbs, relieves congestive headaches.

- Exposing face to steam draws blood to the periphery, relieving headache.

- Prolonged warm immersion baths provide relief.

- Steam baths help in removing toxins through sweat and provide relief for some of the headaches.

- Ice-cold compress or a cold compress, once an hour, kept on the forehead relieves headache due to fever by bringing down the temperature.

- Ice massage to head and spine relieves headache due to high blood pressure.

- Cold or neutral spinal bath, taken regularly, has tonic effect on the nervous system and helps in preventing headache.

- Regular practise of yogasanas, kriyas, pranayama plays a great role in relieving headaches and also in preventing it. Yoganidra and shavasana, which provide a deep sense of relaxation to the mind, are also beneficial, if practiced regularly.

MIGRAINE

Migraine, which afflicts twelve per cent of the world's population, is still a misunderstood phenomenon. Migraine needs no special introduction. There will be a distinctive hammering or throbbing, one-sided headache during an attack, with nausea or vomiting. Only a migraine sufferer knows the severity of the affliction. When it strikes, it stops work, thought and every other activity of the sufferer.

It can take the form of either classical migraine or simple migraine. The classical migraine attack can easily be distinguished from the other by the chain of reactions that characterise it. The troublesome syndrome is preceded by an "aura", which serves as a warning of the headache to follow.

The "aura" may take the form of an uncommon feeling of well-being which alerts the person to expect an attack. The initial symptoms of migraine are, usually, blurring of vision, which may reach its peak in fifteen to thirty minutes and then fade. Normalcy will return in about an hour. Then starts the typical one-sided headache, throbbing in nature, accompanied by nausea and vomiting. The severity of pain ranges from a dull, persistent ache to an unbearable thumping and pounding pain. The pain is triggered off, most of the time, by intense light and high frequency sound.

Simple migraine occurs more frequently than the classical one. It has no aura or any early indications of the impending attack, but all the signs of a typical migraine attack may manifest.

Treatment

1. Preventive Measures

- Treat the underlying precipitating factor, i.e. Indigestion and Constipation, by cleansing the bowels by warm water enema, for the first two to three days.

- Regular practise of yogasanas, kriyas and pranayama improves health and relaxes the body.

- Regular practise of yoganidra, shavasana, progressive relaxation or bio-feedback helps relax the body and the mind, leading to prevention of migraine.

- Other general measures adopted to improve the functioning capacity of the digestive system also help in the treatment of migraine.

2. Before an Attack
- Avoid consumption of condiments, pickles, sugar, tea, coffee, tobacco, alcohol and heavy, spicy food.
- Hot fomentation to the back of the neck is also beneficial.

3. For Relief During Attack
- Head massage, followed by hot foot immersion, cold troma and cold pack help to relieve the symptoms.
- Induced vomiting relieves pressure by emptying the stomach.
- Steam inhalation dilates blood vessels of the face and divert the blood flow, relieving the pain to a certain extent.
- Hot foot and arm bath diverts the blood to the upper and lower limbs and thus helps in relieving the pain.

4. General Measures
- Steam and sauna baths open up sweat pores, eliminate toxins from the body through sweat and clean the internal system.
- Warm water immersion baths, which divert the blood to periphery, if taken for a prolonged period, are beneficial.

Chapter XVIII

Stress and Tension

Stress is a condition that manifests when the individual's adaptive capacity to a given situation is overwhelmed. Any change that requires adaptive behaviour can produce stress. Whatever the level of stress—physical, psychological or emotional—the net result is stress reaction and, which is harmful to the body, leads to diseases, such as Hypertension, Anxiety Neurosis, depression, digestive disorders and Ischaemic heart diseases.

Physical stress is triggered usually by weather, noise, pollution or disease. Emotions like anger, frustration, joy, grief, happiness and embarrassment are psychological stressors.

A certain amount of stress is always desirable because it gives us the required stimulation, drive and motivation to face the challenges of life. This, in fact, is termed as positive stress.

Responses to stress vary from one individual to another. Perhaps the most significant determinant to stress response is one's attitude towards life and the methodology he or she adopts to overcome stressful events.

Treatment

- Diagnosis is the first step. Diagnose the stressful situation first.

- Conscious acceptance of the possibility of the symptoms in relation to stress.

- Adoption of a relaxation technique for proper stress management, such as yoganidra, shavasana, bio-feedback, progressive relaxation and meditation.

- A well-balanced diet and food intake at fixed timings.
- A regular physical exercise, such as walking, yoga and pranayama.
- Cold spinal bath, daily, for thirty minutes.
- Full body massage, once a while, generally relaxes the body, apart from bestowing other benefits.
- Warm water bath, in general, relaxes the system.
- Neutral immersion bath provides relaxation.
- Chest packs and neutral spinal baths, taken regularly, are also beneficial.
- Neutral whirlpool baths, underwater massage steam, sauna and contrast foot baths also prove beneficial.
- Cold foot bath, for thirty to forty-five minutes, relieves tension.
- Setting sensible goals, keeping calm in all situation, cultivating habit of spending time purposefully, and adequate rest and relaxation, all go a long way in preventing stress reaction.

Chapter XIX

Colon Hydrotherapy

The colon or large intestine is about five to six feet long. It is the body's major eliminative organ. The primary function of the colon is to absorb water, electrolytes and vitamins, and to prepare and store faecal waste prior to elimination. From the colon, waste material and toxins move to the rectum and anus for final discharge.

Colon, often with wrong diet, insufficient water intake, lack of exercises, stress and sedentary lifestyle, gets clogged with putrefied matter and over-bacterialisation, leading to many diseases. If it is clogged for longer period, it loses its tone and also the body loses its natural and normal defence mechanism, leading to Constipation. Naturopathy believes that Constipation is the root cause of most of the diseases. Hence, cleaning the colon thoroughly is very important.

In colonic irrigation, pure water is used under controlled temperature and pressure, to wash out the stagnated faecal material and detoxify the colon.

Procedure: The patient is to lie comfortably on a specially-designed table. A sterlilised nozzle is gently inserted in the anus by an expert. The water is slowly infused into the colon through an equipment developed in USA, after a great deal of research. The equipment has auto system in monitoring pressure and temperature. It has one inlet and one outlet pipe, through which clear water is infused and waste water taken out simultaneously. During the time of colonic session, the technician is to freely communicate with the patient so that both pressure and temperature are controlled at a level where the patient is absolutely comfortable. A session usually continues for forty to fifty minutes, consuming about twenty-five gallons (one hundred and twenty-five litres) of warm and potable water, with requisite pressure to flush the entire length of five to six feet of colon.

The colon can be fully cleansed in a series of session, each time, gently removing the toxins and encrusted obstructions. An initial treatment of three sessions is normally recommended. A session can be taken on alternate days. However, in certain cases, doctors may prescribe even four to six sessions. At the end of the second and fourth sessions, a dilution of juice of half a lemon and half teaspoonful of salt in one cup of warm water should be infused through syringe to dissolve the stuck up faecal matter on the walls of the colon, and then released. After a colonic session, patients should go to the toilet to evacuate.

To avoid infection and contamination, extreme care is to be taken. Speculums are disposable, while other items are sterilised. The toilets and the entire system are thoroughly disinfected.

Benefits: Colonic irrigation improves the level of functioning of the whole body. Response to treatment is quicker and more effective after the administration of colonic irrigation. It is beneficial for the patients of Indigestion, Constipation, Obesity, Migraine, Sinus, Asthma, Arthritis, Diabetes, Hypertension, etc. Though there is loss of electrolytes, salts and flora, these can be restored through supplements like oral electrolytes, acidophyllus and proper diet. Patients are advised not to eat two hours before and after colonic irrigation. Patients should preferably take liquid diet like butter-milk, juices, etc. on the day of colonic session.

Contraindication: The treatment is contraindicated in heart problem, Cirrhosis of liver, Hernia, advanced pregnancy, severe Hypertension, ulcerative Colitis, Haemorrhoids, Epilepsy, psychic depression, severe Diverticulitis, etc.

Chapter XX

Acupuncture

Acupuncture is a treatment modality of Chinese origin, dating back five thousand years. The treatment of various diseases by inserting very fine needles into specific points of the body is termed acupuncture. In Latin, *acus* means needle and *punge* means pricking. The whole body is endowed with a number of spots—the acupoints. These points, when stimulated by needles, bring about the cure. Needle stimulation can be given by hand or by electricity. The heating is done by burning a herb, *Artemisia vulgaris*, and the technique is called moxibustion. The two techniques, needling and moxibustion, can be used separately or in combination.

Effects of Acupuncture: When a needle is inserted on the acupoints of the body, it leads to various types of subjective and objective effects. Subjective effects are pain, numbness, soreness, heaviness and distension. Objective effects are analgesia, sedation, immunity improvement and homeostasis. A combination of more than two types of feelings indicates that the needles have been accurately placed and energy is stimulated properly.

In order to find and mark correct location of points, measurement of individual patient's body size is essential. The width of the joint near the patient's thumb is taken as an unit.

According to the traditional Chinese descriptions, twelve paired meridians and two unpaired meridians are present in the body. The twelve paired meridians originate from the internal viscera of the body and are named according to the viscera of origin.

Acupuncture needle: Acupuncture needles are made of various metals, such as gold, silver, copper and steel. Nowadays, the most commonly used needles are of stainless steel, which come in three to four varieties. Needles are available both in disposable and reusable kind.

In the treatment by Acupuncture, it is not only essential to select and locate the points precisely, but also to use appropriate manipulation of the needles in accordance with the nature of the disease and the chosen point. The exact location of each acupoint and its method of use are most important in obtaining maximum benefit in the treatment.

This treatment can be given for twenty minutes everyday, for seven to ten days (one course). For better results, one or two more courses can be taken by giving a gap of seven to ten days.

Acupuncture has been successfully utilised in curing various complicated diseases, including diseases of nerves, muscles, joints, mental depression, heart, digestive system, high blood pressure, Diabetes and respiratory problems. It is also effective in menstrual disorders and in medical emergencies like coma and shock.

In the recent years, acupuncture anaesthesia is one of the most important development which has certain advantages over the modern anaesthesia.

Contraindication of Acupuncture:
- Surgical cases
- Patient receiving drugs for certain diseases. In these cases, particular attention must be paid.
- In the first and last trimester of pregnancy, it is best avoided.
- Haemorrhagic diseases

Acupuncture should always be taken from a qualified Acupuncturist.

Chapter XXI

Miscellaneous Conditions

FEVER

Fever is a warning signal that the body sends out, indicating that something is wrong with the system. Fever is an acute condition and all acute conditions are direct manifestation of the self-cleaning and health-restoring activity of the body. Fever should be allowed to run its natural course in order to have better health once it subsides on its own.

If the fever is suppressed with antipyretics or antibiotics, it will only lead to other chronic diseases. Hence, the best way to treat fever is not to interfere with the body's self-healing process.

Fever is generally accompanied by increased body pains, generalised fatigue, malaise and distaste in the mouth.

Treatment

- Only liquids, such as lime juice, tender coconut water or orange juice should be given, three-four times a day, till the symptoms subside. The patient should be encouraged to drink plenty of water.

- No solid food consumption till fever subsides.

- Warm water enema, early in the morning, during the fasting period, for the first three days, and thereafter, as per the need, till the fasting is discontinued.

- Mudpacks, for fifteen to twenty minutes, two or three times a day.

- Frequent chest pack and cold compress on the forehead.

- Cold sponge bath or cold friction bath is invigorating, and at the same time, brings down the body temperature.

- Rubbing the spine with ice also reduces the temperature.

- Adequate rest and relaxation with light clothing, in a well-ventilated room, are essential.

- Once the temperature comes down and the coating on the tongue reduces, fasting should be discontinued with fresh fruit juices, and later on, with fresh, juicy fruits, raw salads, sprouts and soups. Gradually, one should switch over to normal diet.

ABSCESSES

These are closed cavities containing pus. Abscesses cause pain, occasionally fever, accompanied by chills and malaise.

Treatment
- Fasting to cleanse the internal system.

- Warm water enema, initially, during the fast. Mudpacks to be applied three to four times a day.

- All other measures to improve general health should be employed.

- Bathing the abscess with warm Epsom salt water reduces the pain.

- Ice packs wrapped around the abscess also reduce pain and swelling.

- Application of hot poultice, made of wheat flour paste (prepared by mixing the flour in boiling water), mixed with turmeric powder, packed in a muslin cloth, and wrapped around the abscess overnight, will remove the accumulated pus by next day.

- Fomentation to the abscess and mud application relieve the pain.

- Once the abscess opens up, it should be bathed frequently with warm water to prevent re-infection.

BUNIONS

Bunions form as a result of wearing ill-fitting shoes. If the footwear is too small or too narrow, the big toe joint is forced inwards, resulting in its inflammation and enlargement due to constant pressure and irritation.

Treatment

- Select a footwear that fits properly and whose straight, inner margin does not cause compression on the big toe.
- A pad of cotton kept between the first two toes prevents bunions from forming.
- Stretch the big toe regularly, in correct direction, after removing footwear.
- Warm water Epsom salt bath to the feet is useful in relieving pain caused by the bunion.

BRUISES, STRAINS, SPRAINS AND MUSCLE INJURIES

No matter how healthy one is, it is absolutely impossible to avoid an occasional sprain or a bruise.

Treatment

- Rice principle to be strictly followed.

    R - Rest. Complete rest for twenty-four to forty-eight hours.

    I - Ice packs to the affected area for twenty to thirty minutes, once in every two hours, for twenty-four to forty-eight hours.

    C - Cold compress. Frequent cold compresses reduce bleeding and swelling by constricting the blood vessels.

    E - Elevation of the sprained area reduces swelling.

- Continuous use of cold compresses reduces the flow of blood, and hence, delays healing. Therefore, after twenty-four to forty-eight hours of ice-cold applications, hot applications to be employed on the affected area to restore blood circulation, which will speed up the healing process.
- Employ hot and cold baths frequently.

- In case of bruises or abrasions, intake of foods rich in Vitamin C should be recommended to speed up the healing.
- Cold pack and ice massage, applied to bruises and injured muscles, reduces pain immediately.
- Hot water application, later on, in the form of fomentations or affusions, over the bruises and injured muscles, after first twenty-four hours of ice massage, are often beneficial.

HEAT EXHAUSTION

It usually occurs when the body is exposed to extreme heat, especially when excess clothing is worn while working in closed, badly ventilated rooms. It's symptoms include fainting, cold and damp skin, and feeble or rapid pulse rates, but most cases recover soon.

Treatment
- The patient should be removed to a cool place and given a brisk rubbing with a cloth dipped in cold water.
- Lemon juice with honey added to hot water will provide the energy required and should be given periodically.
- Cold chest pack will stimulate the heart, promoting normal circulation.
- Cold compression on forehead is useful.
- If the body temperature is below normal, then legs should be wrapped with cloth dipped in hot water, with a blanket over it.

HICCOUGH

It occurs due to the spasm of the diaphragm, caused by nervous irritation.

Treatment
- Drink a glass of warm water.
- Fomentation to abdomen and cold compress can relieve pressure on diaphragm.
- Diversion of attention elsewhere.
- Deep breathing.

- Sipping of ice-cold water, slowly.
- Taking a spoonful of honey or sugar stops hiccoughs immediately.

EPISTAXIS (NOSEBLEEDING)

Bleeding from the nose may be due to external trauma, nose picking, nasal infection or drying up of nasal mucosa. Sometimes, the blood drains into pharynx and is swallowed.

Nosebleeding may occur due to blood Dyscrasia, Hypertension, nasal tumors, etc., where before treatment, it is necessary to detect the underlying cause and treat accordingly.

Treatment
- The patient should lie down, slightly lowering his head. Ice-cold compress should be placed over the nose, which will facilitate clotting of blood.
- Avoid blowing the nose.
- Sniffing cold water mixed with lemon juice helps to stop the bleeding.

TOOTHACHE

Toothache is surely one of the most excruciating of pains ever suffered by man. It is often accompanied with swelling.

Treatment
- Fomentation and cold compress to be applied to cheek on the affected side. This reduces inflammation by diverting the blood circulation.
- Brushing teeth, rubbing with salt and gargling, later on, with warm saline water, help to bring down the pain.
- General measures, which improve health and maintain good oral hygiene, provide relief.
- Fasting often helps in controlling secondary infection, and thus, provides relief from pain.

Tips for Healthy Living

MAINTAIN
Water

- Drink one to three glasses of warm/cold water in squatting position after rising from the bed in the morning.
- Drink at least eight to twelve glasses of water everyday, with a frequency of one glass every two hours.

Vital Factors

- Breathe deeply and keep an erect posture always.
- Cultivate the habit of passing bowel motion twice a day.*
- Bathe twice a day with cold/netural water.*
- Pray/meditate twice a day.*

Rest

- After every meal, pass urine, and relax in vajrasana for five to fifteen minutes.
- Sleep on a medium/hard bed with a thin pillow.
- Forget your worries and be relaxed when you go to bed.
- Cultivate the habit of sleeping on abdomen or on the right side.
- Keep at least three hours gap between dinner and bedtime.

Exercise

- Early morning brisk-walk/jog for thirty minutes.

---

* Once in the morning, before sunrise, and once at night.

- Exercise regularly, do asanas, suryanamaskaras, practise gardening, swimming, play games, etc.
- Go for a stroll after dinner, for fifteen to twenty minutes.

Food

- Chew well and eat slowly and calmly.
- Eat according to your hunger, but fill only three-fourth of your stomach.
- Ideal timings for meals are between 9a.m. and 11a.m. and 5p.m. to 7p.m.
- Take only two meals a day (with a gap of about seven hours).
- Use any grains/seeds only after soaking them in water overnight.
- Take dried fruits also after soaking them in water overnight.
- Let one part of your meal consist of cereals and another of vegetables. Do not mix cooked and raw diet. Take raw diet in one meal and cooked in another.
- Use only pure oil having unsaturated fats, such as sunflower or gingili oil.
- Take more of raw food—sprouts, fresh, green, leafy vegetables, seasonal fruits, salads, juices, raw chutney, lemon/honey/water. Prefer butter-milk and curds to milk.
- Cooked food should include whole flour, unpolished rice and gruel. Preferably, use steam-cooked food and soup.

REDUCE/MODERATE

- Salt, sweets, spices, chillies, pulses (dal), ghee, cream, butter, ice cream, cooked food, potato and nuts.
- High heel footwear, weight, strenuous exercise, etc.

AVOID

- Smoking, tea, coffee, alcohol, drugs, soft drinks, tobacco chewing, *paan*, zarda and other bad habits.
- White flour (maida), white sugar, polished rice.

- Non-vegetarian food.
- Tinned/dried/adulterated/coloured/flavoured/synthetic /artificial food.
- Refined/deodorised/bleached/hydrogenated (*vanaspati*) oils.
- Food when in fear, worry, anxiety, and when not hungry.
- Very hot and very cold food.
- Air/water/noise pollution.
- Harmful cosmetics, medicated soaps and creams.
- Drinking water during meals and within half an hour before and upto one hour after.
- Late dinner.
- Heavy meals.
- Late sleeping.
- Sleeping on the left side and on the back.

PRACTISE
- Gargling with lukewarm saline water once a day.
- Wash your eyes with *triphala* water daily in the morning and in the evening, for sparkling eyes.
- Do "vamana dhauti" (kunjal/vomiting) once a week.
- Take enema, if constipated.
- Massage and sunbath, once a week.
- Do gentle massage over palate (roof of mouth) daily.
- Splash water, twice daily, on forehead and eyes, keeping your mouth full of water.
- Spend some time in laughing and singing daily.

PRECAUTIONS
- Wash vegetables and fruits properly before cutting, as they contain pesticides and contaminants.
- As far as possible, eat wholesome fruits and vegetables along with the peel.

ADOPT
- Early to bed and early to rise habit.
- Fasting once every week with juices and adequate water.
- Eat to live, not live to eat.
- Nature cure in case of illness, as well as for good health.

POINTS TO REMEMBER
- Food occupies sixth place in the following requisites for living.
  - Adequate space
  - Pure air
  - Pure water
  - Sunshine
  - Exercise/physical work
  - Food
- Drugs are more dangerous than diseases.
- Those who are regular in food, exercise and sleep/rest, never fall sick.
- Water is the medicine and diet is the drug.
- Fasting is an important factor in any cure.
- Hurry, worry and curry makes a man ill.

POINTS AT A GLANCE
- All healing powers are within your body.
- Nature cure is the safest and the most permanent cure.
- Do not eat if ill, tired, in pain, in a tense state or in a hurry.
- Food taken in sickness feeds the disease, not the patient.
- Drink water half an hour before or one hour after your meals.
- Good health depends on a well-balanced diet and a happy attitude towards life.
- Drugs, tobacco and alcohol are the other poisons that have to be condemned.
- Drink at least eight to twelve glasses of water everyday.

- Keep at least three hours gap between dinner and bedtime.
- Money can buy medicine, not health.
- Nature is rich, let her enrich you.
- A disciplined life makes you live long and happy.
- Tea and coffee may stimulate you for a short time, but ultimately they depress you.
- Yoga has a complete message for humanity. It has a message for the body, the mind and the soul.
- Naturopathy and yoga are like two wheels of a cart.
- Your guide during your period of treatment is your doctor. Have faith in him and your terms for change of diet and treatment.
- Go for a stroll after dinner, for fifteen to twenty minutes.
- Eat according to your day-to-day appetite, but fill only three-fourth of your stomach.
- Avoid smoking, tea, coffee, alcohol, drugs, soft drinks and other bad habits.

Glossary

Abscess: Collection of pus in a cavity.

Appendix: A worm-like structure at the end of the large intestine (colon).

Arthritis Deformans: Rheumatoid Arthritis.

Arteriosclerosis: Hardening of the arteries.

Asthma: A respiratory problem, manifested by breathlessness and wheezing.

Atony: Loss of tone.

Bell's Palsy: Partial paralysis of the face, caused due to oedema (swelling) of the facial nerve. Exact cause unknown.

Bronchitis: Inflammation of the bronchi. May be acute or chronic. Manifested by cough with sputum, difficulty in breathing, etc.

Bunion: Deformity of the foot bone at its junction with the great toe. Friction and pressure of shoes at this point can cause a bursa (sack containing small quantity of fluid) to develop. The bone and bursa are known as Bunion.

Bursitis: Inflammation of bursa.

Cellulitis: Inflammation of connective tissue.

Cranial nerves: Twelve pairs of nerves originating from the brain.

Crepitation: Crackling sound heard in the lungs by means of a stethoscope, usually during lung infections.

Dermatitis: Inflammation of the skin.

Diphtheria: An acute infectional disease involving the upper respiratory tract. Manifested by pain swelling and suffocation in the throat.

Diuretic: Promoting urination.

Dyscrasia: A morbid, general state resulting from the presence of toxic materials in the blood. Word "Dyscrasia" usually refers to abnormality in the blood cells.

Dyspepsia: Indigestion.

Emphysema: A condition where air sacs of the lungs are enlarged and damaged, leading to severe breathlessness.

Eustachian tubes: A canal connecting the pharynx with the middle ear.

Eructation: Belching.

Fallopian Tubes: Two tubes (right and left) opening from the upper part of the uterus, ending near the ovaries.

Fibroid: Benign growth, usually in the uterus.

Gastritis: Inflammation of the mucous membrane of the stomach. Manifested by nausea, vomiting, pain and burning sensation.

Gout: A form of Arthritis, where the big toes are involved.

Gangrene: Death of tissue due to loss of blood supply, followed by bacterial invasion and putrefaction.

Haemorrhage: Consistent, heavy bleeding.

Hyperaesthesia: Extra sensitivity.

Hysteria: A neurosis consisting of instability and frustration, characterised by great emotional excitement.

Inflammation: Reaction of tissues to injury or irritation. Manifested by pain, swelling, heat and redness. Denoted by the term "itis".

Laryngitis: Inflammation of the larynx (organ of voice).

Locomotor Ataxia: Disordered gait and loss of sense of position in the lower limbs.

Lumbago: Pain in the lower back (lumbar) region.

Metritis: Inflammation of the uterus.

Muscle Dystrophy: Degeneration of the muscle.

Myelitis: Inflammation of the spinal cord.

Myositis: Inflammation of a muscle.

Neuralgia: Pain along a nerve route.

Neurasthenia: Denoting lassitude, inertia, fatigue.

Ovaries: Structures which develop the egg (ova), situated on either side of the uterus.

Oophoritis: Inflammation of the ovaries.

Oro-facial: Pertaining to the mouth and face.

Palpitation: Rapid, forceful heartbeat, of which the patient is aware.

Paralysis: Complete or partial loss of nerve functions in a part of the body.

Paraplegia: Loss of nerve function in the lower limbs, including bladder and rectum.

Periodontal: Pertaining to the gums.

Periarthritis: Frozen shoulder.

Peritoneum: The serous membrane in the abdominal and pelvic cavities.

Pharyngitis: Inflammation of the pharynx (cavity at the back of the mouth).

Piles/Haemorrhoids: Dilated veins around the anus.

Pleurisy: Inflammation of the pleura (the membranous covering of the lungs).

Poliomyelitis: A virus infection, which leads to loss of muscle power and flexibility.

Prostate: A small gland at the base of the urinary bladder in males.

Rectum: Lower part of the large intestine.

Reflex: Backward flow.

Salpingitis: Inflammation of the fallopian tubes.

Sciatica: Pain in the distribution of the sciatic nerve (hips, back of thigh, calf, foot).

Sclerosis: Inflammation of the para-nasal sinuses (small cavities in the bones around the nose).

Splanchnic nerves: Nerves supplying to various internal organs.

Spondylorthrosis: Degeneration and inflammation of the intervertebral disc joints.

Spondylolisthēsis: A condition where the vertebra is displaced forward over a lower vertebra.

Subinvolution: Failure of the uterus to return to normal size within the expected time after childbirth.

Tabes: Wasting away.

Tabes Dorsalis: Where the posterior columns of the spinal cord and sensory nerve roots are diseased.

Tendinitis: Inflammation of a tendon (a cord which attaches muscles to the bone).

Testicles: The glandular structures in the scrotum of the male.

Thoracic: Pertaining to the chest cavity (thorax).

Tonsillitis: Inflammation of the tonsils (small bodies on the sides of the back of the mouth).

Toxaemia: A condition where there are toxins in the blood.

Trisums: Spasm in the muscles of mastication (chewing).

Urates: Salts of uric acid. Uric acid is formed by the breakdown of nucleus proteins in the tissues.

Urinary incontinence: Inability to control the evacuation of urine.

Urticaria: Allergic skin reaction, where many pinkish-reddish, itchy rashes errupt.

Uterus: The womb.

Whooping Cough: An infectious disease in children, characterised by attacks of cough, ending with a "whoop".